Also by Tilman Spengler

Lenin's Brain

Spinal
Discord

One Man's
Wrenching Tale of Woe
in Twenty-four
(Vertebral) Segments

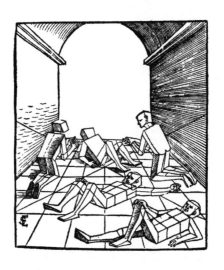

Spinal Discord

TILMAN
SPENGLER

Translated by
PHILIP BOEHM

Metropolitan Books
Henry Holt and Company
New York

Metropolitan Books
Henry Holt and Company, Inc. / *Publishers since 1866*
115 West 18th Street / New York, New York 10011

Metropolitan Books is an imprint of
Henry Holt and Company, Inc.

Originally published in Germany in 1996 as *Wenn Männer
sich Verheben* by Rowohlt Berlin Verlag GmbH

Published in Canada by Fitzhenry & Whiteside Ltd.,
195 Allstate Parkway, Markham, Ontario L3R 4T8

Library of Congress Cataloging-in-Publication Data

Spengler, Tilman.
[Wenn Männer sich verheben. English]
Spinal discord : one man's wrenching tale of woe
in twenty-four (vertebral) segments /
Tilman Spengler : translated by Philip Boehm.—1st American ed.
p.   cm.
ISBN 0-8050-5552-5 (alk. paper)
I. Title.
PT2681.P46W4513   1997
833'.914—dc21   97-19606

Henry Holt books are available for special promotions
and premiums. For details contact: Director, Special Markets.

First American Edition 1997

Designed by Victoria Hartman
Woodcut from *Lessons in Proportion* by Erhard Schoen, Nürnberg, 1534
Drawings after Schoen by Britta Paulich

Printed in the United States of America
All first editions are printed on acid-free paper. ∞

1   3   5   7   9   10   8   6   4   2

To Lena

CONTENTS

Spinal
Discord

First Vertebra

THE NEW LORD

"I am your new Lord," said Pain, by way of introduction. "Henceforth thou shalt have no other god before me." He had no form, only a clarion voice, and a mighty grip that took hold of me just above the buttocks.

Our initial encounter occurred at precisely 7:43 A.M. on a Monday morning. Because I've had to recall it so often, I have a tremendous command of all the details. The prevailing meteorological conditions where I live were well within the seasonal norms. The futon I had been sleeping on for three and a half years had been restuffed just six months earlier.

The previous evening I had spent four hours in a pub with several friends, none of whom detected any visible tension in my appearance. In fact, according to them I had been "pretty well-oiled" as I launched into a colorful catalog of indiscretions committed by a certain notoriously strait-laced editor-in-chief. There was nothing particularly daunting about these anecdotes, nor did the telling cause me any noticeable stress.

I spent those hours in the pub alternately sitting down and standing up. Actually I had spent the whole day both sitting and standing, moving from one desk to another: my study has one for standing and one for sitting, and I go back and forth according to which telephone happens to ring, or depending on where at any given moment I'm feeling particularly uninspired.

And, since this question too is bound to come up, the answer is no: I spent the night alone. So there were no excesses of any kind that might be construed as gymnastically challenging. Of course, anyone acquainted with my love life would have been surprised to learn that there had been. No, I can assure you that all I did before going to sleep was read a few pages of *Pride and Prejudice*, a text one could hardly consider onerous, especially in the paperback edition. And then I woke up, and there was Pain, determined not to let me climb out of bed, or pull on my socks, or lean over the sink, or even think of spending the next several nights with anyone other than Jane Austen.

Pain seemed to know me pretty well; he knew exactly how to counter every move I made to wriggle out of his grasp, and I began to suspect that he might be an old forgotten friend—or, at any rate, a longtime acquaintance. But just because he knew me didn't mean that I knew him. When I was a child, pain was a scraped knee, a teacher's spanking, a bully at recess. Later on it usually came as the result of athletic hubris and went by names like sprained ankle, torn ligament, shin splint, or charley horse—the body's indignant reactions to having been so grossly imposed upon, flare-ups of anger quickly followed by reconciliation.

That kind of pain smacked of something ruddy and robust, of flushed cheeks and sweaty locker rooms. What I experienced on this Monday morning, however, was the harsh, cold sneer of a police interrogator assuring his prisoner that he would not relent until—until what? Aren't I entitled to a phone call? Shouldn't I have a lawyer present? Or else, just let me sign a confession and be done with it!

I tried sticking my tongue out at him. I tried laughing out loud, sarcastically, derisively—it's often the best thing to do in the face of humiliation. Except I couldn't laugh very loud. It hurt.

So I decided to defend myself by resorting to what psychologists call "infantile regression"—though I could care less what they call it if only it had worked. In any event, I was astonished when I realized I was growing older and younger at the same time: I was turning into a doddering toddler. And on the very day I determined to call my doctor, I was reduced to an honest-to-God crawl, and it dawned on me that I might actually be an evolutionary throwback to some phase between tortoises and toads.

My doctor thought less in epochs than in years. Wielding the phrase "Men of your age" like a pair of tweezers, he deftly positioned me in his collection. Then he launched into a lecture on weight loss and injections, warm baths and psychic stress. His voice dispensed a bubbly optimism.

"So what's wrong with me?" I asked, eager to learn the name of my painful condition.

"Diagnoses over the telephone are always a little tricky," my doctor said. "But if you insist upon considering the symptoms you have described, my hunch would be that this is a classic case of chronic LBP."

Hunch! Thank you very much. Still, despite his tasteless, casual manner, I did take a certain comfort in his use of technical language; I read it as an attempt to bond with me, to include me and accept me as one of the initiated. Of course, the abbreviation he used sounded more like the name of some new mutual fund, until it finally struck me, just as I was hoisting myself off the floor: chronic lower back pain.

"Consider yourself unmasked!" I said to Pain after I had finally settled in bed, exhausted. I would have underscored this taunt with a satisfying, scornful laugh, but all I could manage was a wheezy pant.

So round one went to Pain.

Second Vertebra

IN THE COMPARTMENT

For over a hundred kilometers we had been aware that the little girl was the old lady's granddaughter. We also knew they would both be getting off in Würzburg, ever since the conductor had advised them of their best connections. Actually, apart from his uniform there was nothing very conductor-like about the man, with his calculator and cellular phone. In any event this well-accoutred official suggested that "the ladies" take the Randsacker local, "although it would also be possible to catch a special bus operated by the train company"—here there came a flurry of electronic calculation—"which, despite a somewhat later departure time should arrive some . . . twenty-two minutes sooner. But, then again, taking into account the relative comfort of our trains, personally . . ." And so on.

Until that moment the little girl had been concentrating intently on a crossword puzzle evidently devoted to paleontology. She hadn't said a word except to herself, and even then she spoke with absolutely no inflection and without looking up from her notebook: "Extinct order of reptiles" or "hornlike growth." At every word she gave the tip of her pencil a little lick before pressing it to the paper. The men in the compartment would glance up from their newspapers, smiling gently.

The conductor was halfway out the door when the little girl pointed her moistened pencil point at the luggage rack. "And what about our big heavy suitcase?" she asked in an improbably high soprano, her greenish eyes glittering behind her glasses.

The uniformed man spun around, took one look at the suitcase, and replied casually, perhaps jokingly, that "the little lady" had no cause for worry since she was "surrounded by so many gallant gentlemen." Then he turned and walked out with a mysterious urgency, shutting the door behind him. And although it was impossible to tell whether it was due to her question or his reply, the mood in the compartment changed dramatically.

First to react was a man with neatly ironed jeans jutting out from underneath the financial pages. He was sitting right next to the little girl and therefore in a good position to assess the object she had brought into focus with such charming clarity. As he lowered his newspaper, I managed to catch a glimpse of his face: early forties, with ruddy cheeks which had undoubtedly been scrubbed pink when he was little, and which were now kept rosy with musk-scented cologne.

But these same cheeks turned a pale shade of yellow the moment he caught sight of the suitcase. He let his paper drop onto his lap, gripped both armrests of his seat and pushed himself up, less like a passenger rising to retrieve his hat and coat than a gymnast attempting a backward lift above the bar. Keeping his lips pursed and his eyes shut, he swayed his bottom back and forth several times, then sank down again into his seat, melting into the upholstery to form a kind of bas-relief that grimaced and groaned at every unevenness in the rails.

From that point on, the suitcase loomed inside our compartment like a gigantic monster that grew more threatening with every passing kilometer. Its reinforced edges with their black plastic trim seemed to stretch out in all directions, as if a giant octopus were spreading its tentacles, distracting us from such urgent matters as the decline of the lira, the pros and cons of twelve-cylinder engines, or the future of Hong Kong.

Where once had existed the world, now there was suddenly only this suitcase, mocha brown with double latches, gleaming, viscid, omnipresent.

Meanwhile, freedom was rapidly racing by outside the smoked windows as vineyard nestled up to vineyard and a calm afternoon sun studied its reflection on windshields and wrinkled fish ponds. The little girl asked herself a question about the Pleistocene epoch.

The man sitting to my right had been poring over a book that, from what I could tell, consisted entirely of graphs and tables. Every now and then he would scribble a question mark or an exclamation point next to one of the black or gray columns. But then, just as we emerged from a tunnel, the grandmother glanced at her wristwatch, and the pen slipped out of my neighbor's hands and onto the burgundy-colored industrial carpeting that covered the floor of our compartment.

The table-and-graph man was on the verge of bending over when he thought better of it and began instead to lift himself out of his seat. In doing so he performed a series of screwlike twists, which, according to the degree of turn, brought him alternately close to my ear and further away. After two extreme twists, he reached up and grabbed hold of the luggage rack as if it were a lifeline in a roaring sea. Finally he was standing fully upright, so that his forehead was level with the suitcase. He briefly shut his eyes, then left the compartment.

"That man dropped his pen," the little girl told her grandmother.

And what about the fellow sitting directly across from me? His short, stocky build and sparse hair made him look like a former middleweight boxing champ.

Was he feigning sleep? Or was he preparing to follow the example of the human screwdriver?

No, the champ simply pulled a silver flask from his breast pocket, uncorked it with his teeth, and held it up to his lips—just as he had done when we left Nürnberg. A few long swigs, a happy burp, and then he gently closed his eyes and fell asleep, while the grandmother snuggled the little girl protectively under her arm.

All of a sudden I myself was overcome by an unexpected coughing fit and, sadly, had to leave the compartment.

So exactly what happened when the suitcase pulled into Würzburg, only the two ladies know for sure.

Third Vertebra

STRESS STRUCTURE SHIFT

While I have yet to abandon all hope, I am surrounded by hell: cyclists swishing down the sidewalk, cursing my tortoise pace; skateboarders hurtling past, taking me for just another pole in their ruthless slalom; a moving man hauling a refrigerator on his back, shooing me out of his way.

I have twice negotiated the hundred meters from my cramped apartment to the palatial "Fitness Studio," where, as part of my rehabilitation, I learn to swing my arms and twist my pelvis. However, as a result of my condition I can no longer appear in public unmolested; my shuffling gait has become the focus of unwelcome social attention. Those who don't simply shove me out of the way shrink back in horror, fearful that I might suddenly hit them up for spare change.

But whereas a bona fide bum can count on at least a modicum of sympathy, our society allows no pity for those lumbar sufferers whose pain is "nonspecific" in the eyes of the medical establishment. Perhaps the label "nonspecific" itself is to blame for the general public scorn. Whatever the cause, the truth is that for every case of so-called specific back pain—the wounded veteran, for example—there are two of us men whom God has, in the Psalmist's words, "beaten with a rod of iron." We are the groaning majority, the backbone of the movement, nameless Atlases bearing the burden of the world.

At night, in the hours when I used to sleep or pursue other pleasures, I now lie in bed, acutely awake, and pass the time reading about my fellow sufferers. The titles alone are enough to show how grim an undertaking this can be: *Back Pain, the Occupational Health Hazard* (subtitled: *Promoting the Practice of Prevention*). While I cannot count the author of this particular study as a personal acquaintance, I have no doubt that he is one of us, since, as I have discovered in my long experience, there is inevitably a connection between unmitigated pain and an unpolished style.

I was poring over this excruciating treatise—all the time careful to maintain proper posture for reading in bed—when suddenly I came across the concept "stress structure shift," which seemed to articulate what I had always suspected: namely, that we are living on the threshold not only of a new millennium but of a new era.

Oswald Spengler examined the social structure of Western civilization and concluded it was doomed to decline. Sigmund Freud examined the psychic structure of his contemporaries and concluded that the whole bourgeois world was headed for a breakdown. Each was right in his own way, but actually anybody could have come up with the same prognosis without all that delving into sub-conscious drives and cataloging symptoms of decadence. You don't need to be a Darwin to plot the trajectory of human evolution, from *Homo erectus* to the contemporary *Homo sapiens* and realize that we are approaching the end of the upright gait, at least among the males of the species.

Let's take my comrades-in-suffering from the gym. It's impossible to tell by looking just what glorious heights these men had attained before their mighty downfalls. Only a few years ago these same hunchbacks may have been daredevil acrobats, heroes of track and field, the limberest of limbo dancers. And today? They are flummoxed by the prospect of sitting in on a board meeting where the chairs are anything less than ergonomically sound. Feigning politeness, they are quick to fend off invitations to take a spin in a low-slung sports car. The only vaults they tackle are at the bank, and the idea even of a slow fox-trot sends shivers up their crooked spines.

So what's to blame? As I said, I've read almost everything there is to read on the subject, and I can refute just about every hypothesis. First, the argument that back pain is the inevitable consequence of this generation's failure to handle the transition from physical toil to sedentary tedium . . . Fiddlesticks! The men at my sports club never toiled in their lives, apart from the rare athletic push or the occasional airport marathon. Nevertheless, once upon a time they stood erect.

Then there are the heavily footnoted, socio-psychological whodunits, whose authors point their collective incriminating finger at that archvillain, psycho-lumbar stress.

Balderdash! All the reliable medical sources maintain that, in the hour of his greatest stress, Napoleon suffered not from back pain but from acute gastritis (the result of an undercooked goose). And when you consider how much time he spent in the saddle—well, I'm sure a contemporary emperor would press into service an entire company of chiropractors. Nor did Casanova—yes, I realize that's a different matter, and I'll come back to it later—ever find that his performance suffered due to job-related anxiety. Do you think Churchill, who certainly had his share of stress, ever complained of back pain? Or Gandhi? Or Mao Zedong?

Obviously each of these men suffered his pressures and paid the price for his success, though in a different currency than back pain. But if psychological stress is not to blame for this shift of epochal proportions, what is?

Sadly, science has thus far failed to solve the problem. We must therefore look to other means to untangle this mystery.

Fourth Vertebra

AT THE HEALER'S

"Of things that exist," mused the taxi driver, "some exist by nature, some from other causes." A hill loomed before us and he shifted into a lower gear. "And some things happen through their own initiative," he added, after he had mastered the hill. We were driving through the south of Austria, on our way to a healer who lived near the Slovenian border.

There is a special relationship between cabbies and passengers prone to back pain. Any taxi driver worth his wheels is quick to size up clients according to how they climb into his vehicle—from the limber to the arthritic to the sciatical. Incidentally, medical researchers seriously interested in investigating the phenomenon described in the previous chapter as "stress structure shift" would be well advised to collect data from these learned authorities, who always keep a finger on the pulse of the times while their hands are on the steering wheel. The most prominent in the field can be recognized by the wooden beads draped over the driver's seat like a medieval coat of mail.

My driver must have been a specialist of international renown, for he even covered the passenger seat with such beads. So I was happy to hear his positive opinion of my healer: "The man's strong as a bear, with a good head on his shoulders, and when his mother helps out he's the best there is. The two of them together are a pair of genuine miracle workers."

The driver, it turned out, had previously taken his own complaints to an Indian chiropractor in Graz, a Chinese acupuncturist in Burgenland, a female herbalist from Salzburg, the chief surgeon in the Klagenfurt Hospital, and finally to a deaf Sufi from Iran who was living in Vienna. "And all the while I kept lighting a candle to Saint Nicodemus—that's really supposed to work well, especially when it hurts right here, just above your ass."

Back sufferers are the true representatives of ecumenical thought in our time. They pay homage to diverse gods in diverse ways. Pain leads them to cross borders of space and time; it erases boundaries between science and religion; it harkens back to a time when lumbago was thought to be caused by witchcraft. Of course such reasoning was very misogynist, but CLBP is very much a male problem, and where else would so many traumatized males direct their wrath and indignation? Inexcusable though it may have been, there was something genuine about the reaction, and something appealingly simple about a time when religious rite and medical ritual shared the same intrinsic value. I was determined to give my healer a fair trial.

On the other hand, I was becoming less and less kindly disposed toward the local highway department. Austrian roads are known for their wide gouges and hidden potholes, the legacy of heavy farm equipment. They are littered with organic matter and the wreckage of heavy tires that appear out of nowhere and demand rapid reaction and deft maneuvering on the part of the driver, not to mention the saddle-sore passenger.

This particular road required that I hover above my seat, cushion my right shoulder against the window, and distribute my weight by hanging on to the hand grip, so that I could respond to every painful bump with a smooth, balancing pelvic tilt.

Even so, our encounter with a sizable tree branch caused me to pronounce a hissing curse on the local highway department. My driver didn't even have to check his mirror to deliver his diagnosis: *"Iliolumbalis."* His use of Latin sounded both reverent and imploring, like an urgent intercessory prayer.

"Iliolumbalis" was exactly what the doctor with the rosy face had mumbled as he directed me into a special cylindrical apparatus designed to provide the trained observer, fitted with the proper optical equipment, a true and very intimate picture of the patient's condition. The victim is shoved like a cigar into a metal tube, stark naked, and the machine begins to gently rotate, so that no telltale sign will escape detection. The lens resolves the body into hundreds of black-and-white snapshots of muscle and fiber and bone, reducing the object under scrutiny to a mere biological organism. In the end there is nothing to prove that this same body is also the vessel of a human

soul, one admittedly mired in flesh and prone to sin but nevertheless immortal and worthy of love, particularly when it is struggling to regain composure—as mine was—in the rear seat of a Toyota rocking and bumping down a rainy country road in Carinthia at 80 kilometers an hour.

By the way, *iliolumbalis* is the name of a tiny muscle in the lower back that happens to be particularly inclined to cramping. The doctor with the rosy cheeks had explained all that to me in Munich, but since he had deduced from my chart that I hold an advanced degree, he spoke not of cramps but of coordinated occupational neuroses, contractions of varying intensity, and relapses of the prolapsed intervertebral disc. He also made a very serious, almost puzzled face when he suggested I see a therapist—"someone you can trust." He must not have thought that description applied to him, since he left before I could ask him for a name.

"It sets in at around thirty, and it's all downhill from there . . ." was how my driver phrased his diagnosis. "By the way, see that house over there? That's where your man lives." He pointed his gloved right hand at a villa on top of a small hill. If I didn't know we were at the Slovenian border I would have thought myself in Tuscany: the driveway was lined with cypress and oleander, and above the villa rose a slender tower, dramatically lit with a pale yellow spotlight. I thought of Crusaders and Saracens, a blissful Arcadia and the fount of mysterious Eastern healing arts, and I was quite surprised to discover that my healer's waiting room reeked of vinyl.

Of course vinyl doesn't really reek, although it looks

like it ought to, and it does tend to capture whatever smell wafts its way, especially in waiting rooms. This particular aroma seemed composed of gastric acid, cold sweat, and pus. To that bouquet I added a hint of wet wool, since there had been no place to hang my coat, apart from a row of crucifixes—and I certainly didn't want to do anything that might jeopardize my chances of being cured. I also noticed that the other patients—all of whom were bent and bowed—were holding on to their coats, even though the heat was streaming through the floor vents. Evidently this was a place where all suffering was kept under wraps.

Thus I felt like a very sweaty cross-country skier by the time I entered the examining room. This room was completely bare, except for two plaster statues of the Virgin Mary, a wardrobe, and a horizontal bar designed for upper-level gymnastics. When I began to unbutton my coat, the healer waved at me to stop, as if I had been about to commit some indecent act.

"*Musculus iliolumbalis,*" he said. "Please step up to the apparatus."

Why was it, I asked myself, that to acquire the same diagnosis in Germany you first had to be twirled around stark naked in a cigar tube, whereas near the southern border of Austria a cabdriver's ear or a healer's mere glance at your wool coat was sufficient?

The instrument of torture known as the horizontal bar was originally designed to separate the true gymnasts from the false ones, those predestined for everlasting athletic acclaim from those doomed to eternal physical damnation. For the nonspecific back sufferer, the mere sight of one is enough to provoke a double despair, as he is invariably confronted not only with his current inadequacy, but with all his previous deficiencies as well.

I was already preparing my full confession when the healer commanded me to hold on to the bar and hang there. He then grabbed one of my legs and started swinging it back and forth like a madman. As I am by no means slight of stature, I was not the least bit surprised to soon hear this heavy man huffing and puffing. I was a little taken aback, however, when a piercingly thin voice began intoning *Ave Maria*. There, right behind me, was the healer's mother, on her knees.

"That'll do it," said her son, relieved. He burrowed his left ear in my coat, gave my right boot a twist, and repeated, "That'll do it!"

The mother halted her prayer and, like her son, placed her ear over the spot where, underneath several layers of wet wool, was lurking my *musculus iliolumbalis*. "Not yet! That won't do it!" she replied sternly and picked up with her *Ave Maria* exactly where she had broken off.

After he had jerked my legs around a little more, with just as much vigor if somewhat less vim, the healer again stopped and proclaimed triumphantly: "That'll do it!"

The mother checked her son's handiwork a second time. "That'll do it," she confirmed, "at least for now. Of course the aching will come back. Maybe in months, maybe in years. But until it does, you'll be able to sit up straight again, in any car and at any desk." She crossed herself as if she had just been speaking about the devil and then vanished behind a glass door. I felt so healed I thanked her with a deep bow.

"Genuine miracle workers," said the taxi driver, "him with his muscles and his old lady with her ear! I know somebody in Zagreb, too, this old Bosnian who uses iron rods. Dirt cheap. So next time . . ."

That evening I undressed without a hitch, and climbed into the shower with great agility and dignity. I believe I even mumbled a prayer of thanksgiving.

Fifth Vertebra

SCRUNCH

I'm not so young anymore. A few years ago, when the surprise guest I call "Scrunch" wrenched his way into my life, I was pretty certain that before long I'd be able to retire his portrait alongside those of some other old friends such as Lust or the twins Booze and Cigarettes.

Although these earlier guests could change their form at will, they were always easy to recognize—and, more important, they invariably announced their coming. Never very loudly, but perceptibly enough for the trained ear.

In this respect Scrunch was different. He cast no shadow, he made no noise. Not even Boris, my Jack Russell terrier, could sense his coming.

Initially I treated him with the same courtesy I show all my guests, at least on their first visit. But Scrunch proved a pretty finicky houseguest, with a constant hankering for salves and radiant heat, though when it came to injections he was inconsistent: sometimes he liked them, sometimes he didn't. He would have nothing what-soever to do with pills and went out of his way to avoid any physical contact. He was so picky, in fact, that I be-gan to suspect he was really nothing more than a snooty old snob.

As I said earlier, Scrunch took to showing up without notice, as if it were entirely his decision when would be a good moment to visit. And he had the obnoxious habit of entering without knocking—at least not on the door. More often than not he'd creep up behind me, tap me on the spine, and shout, "Guess who!" I would scrunch over in pain—hence the name—and remain in a foul mood for the rest of his visit.

Nor did he ever indicate how long he intended to stay. At the same time, in his relentless narcissism he insisted I drop whatever I was doing and spend all my waking mo-ments with him, so that for days I'd have to limit my movements to a very few motions, all devoted exclusively to Scrunch. Now, I realize that every visitor has his quirks, but his were adding insult to injury. Admittedly I'm no longer the super-supple athlete I once may have been, the strapping man whose muscular torso—if mem-ory serves me correctly—was the cause of many an admir-ing female glance and fluttering heart, but still, a little consideration, please.

Actually it was only later that I realized just how un-couth this Scrunch really was. At first I was convinced there was a method to his rudeness, since he chose to visit me three times at exactly 7:33 P.M. on three particularly foggy autumn evenings. But then when he showed up during the summer, in the middle of one of our all-too-frequent record-breaking heat waves, I was forced to abandon this hypothesis and accept the fact that this devil struck whenever and wherever the spirit moved him.

Actually it's misleading to call him a houseguest. In fact, he's also visited me very far from home—my professional curiosity takes me to the most isolated areas—in wet savannahs as well as arid mountains. Over time I have learned that no terrain is too rugged, no location too remote to deter Scrunch from dropping in.

Evidently he felt a longing for me, which, the more I knew him, the less willing and able I was to requite. But he has also proven somewhat fickle in his affections, occasionally allowing whole months to pass without a sign—to my great relief. Unfortunately, he's never told me how long he planned to be absent any more than he's warned me how long he planned to stay. So when I finally realized that he had no intention of mending his ways, I decided to negotiate a pact.

"Hey, Scrunch!" I shouted the next time he chose to surprise me, my voice brimming with feigned jocularity. "I'm sorry it's come to this but I'm afraid we're going to have to stabilize our relationship. My professional life is suffering, and so is my male pride and self-respect. I've always been known for being quick to take a stand, on any issue, but this public scrunching is something else. If all you wanted to do was visit me at home, it would be one thing; I could prepare for that, but the way things have gotten . . ."

"I like things just the way they are," Scrunch answered sullenly and disappeared.

What I wanted to propose to Scrunch that morning, when he stomped off so testily, was a period of separation. Dr. N. had assured me it was a perfectly viable method, not only for married couples but for all other relationships as well. The partners create some distance between themselves, and then see what happens.

I therefore decided to spend the next two months at the hot volcanic springs in Abano, Italy. I realize that Italy has resorts that are more beautiful, but what I was after was solitude, and, of course, a longer period of separation from Scrunch. And though he seemed to hound me wherever I went, I had already noticed a distinct disaffinity on his part for sulphur. (I mentioned this partly to defend myself in advance against any allegations that I might be inclined to demonize my antagonist.)

I checked into the hotel and a strangely stooped porter watched as I carried my trunk up several flights of stairs to my room, which had a splendid view of the street. After the man had rubbed his back, taken my tip, and closed the door, I plopped down on the bed. The mattress gave way beneath me like a soft, fluffy cloud, and at that moment the wardrobe door flew open with a gigantic groan.

"I like things just the way they are," said Scrunch, by way of greeting.

Sixth Vertebra

MOVE FOR MOVE

At the end of our consultation, the ortho-pedic specialist with the bright birthmark running up his left nostril imposed a number of restrictions on my move-ments. "Excessive zeal," he said, "can make you prone to cramps, which can lead to complications, particularly when it comes to, well, you know what I mean."

"Well, you know what I mean" wouldn't have surprised me coming from a schoolmarm or an elderly nurse, but it seemed ridiculous for a professor of medicine to resort to a euphemism like that. At least he managed to flash me a salacious smile before saying goodbye.

Even without his warning it was already clear to me that I would have to be on my guard that night with the young art student who had invited me over, ostensibly to rid me of certain hang-ups in my attitude toward art: "You and your inflexible worship of the original." She herself seemed flexible in every way, especially in her language, which was so elastic I often had trouble understanding what she was saying.

Men with my affliction must analyze in advance every gesture and tug, every gentle push and pull of arms or hips or thighs, and take the necessary prophylactic measures against their possible harmful effects. And for most of us there is no action which entails as much bending and stretching as that act which unites lovers in the physical and spiritual fulfillment of their passion. A worldly connoisseur of art, as I had billed myself, in particular would be expected to demonstrate a considerable amorous repertoire, having had the benefit of instructive erotic masterpieces—from ancient petroglyphs to cutting-edge videos, with their rich variety of positions ranging from the perfectly prone to the fully erect. He would also be expected to negotiate the successful transition from one position to the other deftly, elegantly, boldly—with no sign of pain or stress.

The only men who truly understand what skill, what intense concentration this requires are those who know the stiff humiliation of being unable to untie their shoes, no matter how hard they push, how painfully they shriek, how colorfully they curse at attempt after failed attempt. Only the less-than-limber truly recognize what artistry it takes to separate the admired object from her clothing; only they can understand the necessity of planning and the need to disguise the planning as play. Only they can fully appreciate the degree of dexterity lurking behind the seemingly simple handling of hooks and buttons, buckles and zippers.

The art student sighed as my index finger slid down her neck onto the softly rising knoll of her shoulder. "Where I'm beginning to make a name for myself"—her name, incidentally, was Sophie—"is with my work on the Barbizon school and the *pleinairistes*."

I thought of women in shimmering dresses so airy that a breath was all it took to blur fantasy and reality. My finger caught on an elastic band.

"I saw a wonderful exhibit about six months ago," I said, continuing our intellectual foreplay, "called 'Touch of Twilight.'" I launched into a detailed description of the paintings as my thumb joined my finger in determining what manner of object I had encountered.

As I talked, images from the exhibit raced through my mind: discarded veils, unbraided hair, flowing garments unknotted and untied. A third finger had joined the others; I was straining not to show strain. And this was only the tip of the iceberg; if we continued on our present course I would have to address certain significant personal problems, sooner or later. But I stuck stubbornly to the *Barbizonistes*.

"In fact I once made a bid on an original Daubigny"— here I succeeded in loosening the elastic band enough to allow me to proceed with my topographical survey. The further I explored, the more desire began to cloud my reason, and the more muted was the little voice that kept whispering to me: "Make sure your thoracic vertebrae stay properly aligned for full lumbar support."

"Collecting," proclaimed my companion of the flexible speech, "is nothing but a frustrated denial of possibilities." She casually removed my fingers, as if all they had done was straighten her collar. Then she stood up and said, "Let's move over there."

"Over there" meant the back of her narrow apartment, which was dimly lit with two black candles. But even that was enough for me to see that my fears were justified: her bed was devoid of all possible handholds. The two wooden sculptures at its head were mere phallic ornament and of no practical use whatsoever. The rack of knobs, on the other hand, where she had draped various blouses, looked much more trustworthy, but it was permanently affixed to the far wall and at best could be considered only in case of emergency—a case I sincerely dreaded.

Heavy of heart, I recalled the chaste Hollywood films of my youth, in which the couple separated outside the bedroom before reappearing on either side of a carefully turned-down bed, which was divided into two separate but equal halves. The partners were dressed in a cream-colored negligée and freshly pressed pajamas: the woman presented herself as a gift which required little or no unwrapping; the only thing that might need removing were the man's glasses. Because he could lower himself onto his side of the bed at his own pace, the upright man could rest assured that his spine would be lowered safely to the prone position, according to the rules of ergonomic protocol, which as everybody knows delivers a gain in lumbar comfort of over sixty-six percent.

Of course in Sophie's boudoir it was impossible to even think of relaxation. The situation demanded bold moves and a firm grasp of more than art history, and the inevitable consequences would simply have to be borne with dignity.

"Don't let your energy disseminate the aura," whispered the rising star of *pleinairisme*, as she lowered a tousle of red curls onto a pitch-dark silk pillow. I didn't bother to unravel what she meant, focused as I was on undoing what she was wearing.

This garment came close to what my grandparents would have called "long johns," except it was mauve, and contemporary fashion prefers to call it a "bodysuit." The nether flap of the bodysuit is fastened by means of snaps, which are usually under significant tension, since the cut of the bodysuit is designed not only to cover but also shape the lower body. I mention this not in order to commit an indiscretion; I am simply warning the uninitiated about the pain these metal snaps can inflict when they are unloosed and pop open and whack you on the fingertips—like so many electric shocks. Even more important, however, is the fact that in order to unfasten your lover's bodysuit you must first perform a full-fledged vertical pelvic tilt. And herein lies the problem for the spinally challenged Don Juan; he knows that such reckless tilting may precipitate a reversal that will quickly transform his anticipated conquest into a drawn-out and very likely unsuccessful siege.

"See, you're trapped by your own oculocentrism," Sophie chided me gently when she noticed my hesitation. Her voice purred with sympathy and understanding.

Many great painters show human subjects in moments of extreme passion, their faces and bodies twisted in rapture. And the greatest among them have been able to extend their vision inward, to discern and portray the human soul in its quest to escape its mortal confines, in its striving for oneness, serenity, unmitigated bliss. How would they see me, I wondered. How would they paint my body, racked with pain, and still desperately, passionately, and wordlessly trying to communicate to one of their most charming pupils that such oneness is an unattainable ideal for those burdened—as I was—by a lifetime of postural sin?

How it came to pass that the admirably vaulted stomach of the Hagia Sophia suddenly gleamed as vividly as the misty moon described in the Chinese poem does not belong here. Suffice to say it was not without recklessly ignoring my doctor's warnings and, consequently, not without the complications he had cautioned me to avoid.

Sophie rolled over and switched off her nightlamp before treating me to another penetrating observation: "You know," she whispered, "seduction is both the surmounting of distance and the approach of loss." As she drifted off to sleep, another voice began to whisper in my ear: "For I your Lord am a jealous God . . ."

MEN OF MUSCLE

"The human male is a deep vessel of pain," I thought the next morning, after the aching in my lower iliac muscle had mostly faded. Western literature is silent about the *musculus iliopsoas*, although it is undoubtedly responsible for more dramatic situations than Helen's smile, Desdemona's handkerchief, and all the promissory notes in the entire repertory of Russian opera. This is the muscle that bends the hips—or doesn't bend them, or sometimes bends them in painful protest.

It's true that *musculus iliopsoas* doesn't sound very mellifluous, neither in Latin nor any other language. And whereas phrases such as *"che gelida manina"* and even "by the sweat of your brow" have a certain lyrical resonance, it's hard to see the poetry in *"iliopsoas,"* and I'm afraid no epic will ever begin: "Sing, O Muse, of my iliac / For something's wrenched it out of whack."

The fine arts, however, are not afraid to rush in where poetry and opera fear to tread. Sculptors and painters are undeterred by names such as "femural adductor."

"Maybe you'll feel better," said Sophie, who visited me that afternoon, "if you can bask in the aura of some originals." And with that she rose effortlessly from my orthopedically adjustable lumbar support chair and led me to the museum. I was happy to get out, the more so as Sophie's sophisticated remarks were beginning to wear a little thin, and at the museum at least I wouldn't be the exclusive focus of her wit.

A stray titmouse was perched on a lamppost in front of the entrance. She turned her tufted head toward us and called out in her high, nasal titmouse-voice, "Peter! Peter!" We left her on the lamppost and went inside.

How we see art is a function of experience as much as sensitivity: after all, the victim of an automobile accident looks at a wrecked car very differently than the unlicensed pedestrian, and the confirmed alcoholic does not view the bottle the same way as the teetotaler. So it's not surprising that certain genres of painting speak to back sufferers more strongly than others. Still lifes of flowers, or of sausage and cheese, for example, are of mild interest at best; the same applies to many seascapes as well as most Madonnas. Certain detailed battle scenes, on the other hand, tend to attract our attention. But our true passion is reserved for works that show whole groups of muscles, straining under stress or play, painted in colors ranging from eggshell white to bloodred. To be effective, these pictures must be anatomically correct and of sufficient size to inspire awe.

Unerringly I steered us to a room full of exactly such paintings. In one corner an elderly lady was addressing a circle of people who had signed up for the guided tour.

"The muscular type," she read from a slim brown volume, "is inclined to be shorter and broader of stature, with large bones and no fat." To a man, her male listeners sucked in their guts and straightened their backs. "This is because as the fleshy muscles grow," the woman read on, unmoved, "they form a densely packed mass which crowds out all room for fat."

Was Leonardo da Vinci thinking about drawing technique when he wrote those lines, or was he reminiscing about his once youthful body, recalling a time when his own muscles left no room for any fat?

"Notice the transparency with which these bodies are portrayed," our guide went on, standing in front of a huge canvas of a crashing Goliath. "Look at the play of light and shade. Each successive tone in the scale conveys a different degree of strength. And please pay particular attention to the circulatory system. See how strong the muscle fiber looks, and how the veins stick out along the calf. These figures are very majestic and very masculine, yet"—the woman struggled with her text a moment—"yet they are, nevertheless, also surprisingly lithe and limber."

She herself was rather bony and brittle. Tintoretto would never have put her in the foreground, and Boucher, if he'd painted her at all, certainly wouldn't have posed her naked form on a plush divan. Perhaps Leonardo might have shown some interest in her, but that's not very likely either.

I turned to Sophie for her pronouncement, but her eyes were glued to two muscle men grimly smashing marble columns.

"Ecce homo!" she mumbled, in a voice that seemed to mix rapture and ridicule. "Behold the real man, the embodiment of enticement, loudly proclaiming his appeal!"

Her irony I could understand, but I had no idea what Sophie found so "enticing." No one who's ever had to wear an elastic girdle to support his lower back can possibly see anything enticing about the smashing of marble columns. Nor would he be able to recall a time when he did, despite what anyone says about memory's tendency to glorify. And here we come to the real reason why back sufferers are so drawn to certain paintings: it's not that we wish to feel diminished in the face of powerful men hoisting fleshy nymphs and spiriting them away on their shoulders, or strangling slimy black sea serpents with their bare hands. On the contrary, we are simply looking back, chastened, regarding our own past excesses from a pious distance, just as Tannhäuser looked back upon Venusberg, or as a reformed gambler might pause before a casino, or as Saint Francis might behold a hunting party.

"Don't tell me you don't feel any regrets or yearnings." Sophie looked at me quizzically. "Oh, I see," she went on, reading my thoughts. "Just middle-aged resignation, with more than a tinge of self-righteousness?" She turned away and started ogling some bleeding Titan.

Even the guide seemed to be mocking the men in her group, as if she had concluded they were all a pack of wimps and wannabes, men who had tried out for the role of Atlas or Hercules but didn't get the part.

Her scorn was effective, too. Most of the men appeared embarrassed or discomfited. Some were probably even foolish enough to let self-doubt gnaw away at their self-esteem: "What do these guys have that I don't?" Now, I strongly disapprove of censorship, but women really shouldn't be allowed to see pictures like these. Even healthy men should probably be prohibited from doing so; after all, they might get ideas that would completely confound the evolutionary process.

By the time we left the museum a gray twilight had enveloped the roofs of the houses. The titmouse looked at us and sang out "Peter! Peter!" in an indignant voice, then quickly flew off the lamppost and disappeared from sight.

Eighth Vertebra

TARZAN

I was surprised when the film producer asked me to collaborate on a screenplay about Tarzan. Of course, I would have been even more surprised if he'd asked me to play the title role, but he didn't.

It was a bright summer morning; I was working on a commission, sort of a "travel/adventure" piece on the people of the Dong, a tribe presumably living somewhere in southwestern China. The director of a middle-sized travel agency wanted to entice customers with the possibility of making contact with these "elusive, peaceful people." I mention the size of the company in order to give a sense of the size of the commission, which definitely ruled out any eyewitness accounts. Travel to China is expensive to begin with, travel to the tribal areas of the southwest all the more so, and as I know from experience, the cost to the spinal column can be exorbitant. My local library, however, which boasts a remarkably rich collection of anthropological materials, may be easily reached on foot and is equipped with very respectable reading desks and slanted chairs designed to support the muscles that tilt the pelvis, thus making for a safe, upright posture. And if my longings for the sights and smells of southwestern China grew absolutely unbearable, I could always stop in at the library's cafeteria, where the size of the pots and the mystery of their contents called to mind the roadside kitchens in the Guangxi province.

But what does all this have to do with Tarzan? Nothing except the coincidence in time, the fact that the producer called just as I was in the middle of a touching scene in which a "virtually toothless" village elder complains at length about how his people are suffering because they feel unequal to their ancestors. No longer can they perform the ancient rituals—no longer can they uproot the seven bamboo clumps at the Festival of the Moon all in one pull, with nary a wince or groan.

The scene itself was loosely based on some even looser sources, but my account of their suffering was, I thought, sufficiently sincere. In fact, as I strained to picture the ancient ritual in all its backbreaking difficulty, I began to feel the twinge of an empathic reaction. So I was happy when the phone gave me a chance to stretch.

The caller had an unctuous voice that was too slippery to pin down by age or by region. But the jargon he used left no doubt as to his profession, as he rattled off expressions like "preproduction," "script doctoring," "final takes," and—here's where I came in—"some really decent dialogue."

"For all I know," I responded, after pausing just enough

to show lukewarm interest but not unbridled enthusiasm, "Tarzan may well have been a linguistic genius, at least when it came to primate communication, but I'm afraid dialogues such as 'Tragu?'. . .'Ungawa!' are a little beyond my abilities. And that famous elephant yodel—that would be hard to improve upon."

It should be obvious by now that, as with the people of the Dong, whose fate I was on the verge of inventing, here too I had only a vague idea of what I was talking about.

When I was a boy, Tarzan comic books were absolutely taboo in our house, and I dread to think what my parents would have done if they'd caught me spending my allowance to see a movie where some half-naked man went swinging on jungle vines over treacherous quicksand, always to land at the feet of a grateful buxom blonde. Instead I had to content myself with the myths and legends my parents deemed proper boyhood models of heroism. I'm sure it was on account of this unfulfilled longing that I didn't hang up right away.

"Actually . . . all I'm asking is whether your schedule might permit you to accept a potential offer at some later date," the voice slithered on, "but since you're so familiar with the subject, I don't have to remind you that Tarzan was really the scion of an old English noble family who ultimately took his seat in the British House of Lords. At least in the original version by Edgar Rice Burroughs. But for now why don't I go ahead and transfer you to someone in our business office who can fill you in on the financial details."

I could see the snare beginning to tighten, but this bothered me less and less the more I envisioned the ridiculous sums of money the film industry supposedly lavishes on its writers. "Why not," I told myself, and decided to milk the moment further.

"Of course, they don't speak any more coherently in the House of Lords," I parried, "than Tarzan did before he met Jane. . . . But seriously, I'm not sure if I can interrupt my current work on the people of the Dong. Southwest China. Matriarchal society, male cults. Very complicated stuff, and very exciting."

In my heart of hearts I realized I had already been "bought," or at least, as they say in the business, "optioned." So when a resolute female voice phoned the next afternoon and suggested several possible times for a preliminary discussion of the script—which they really wanted "yesterday"—I opted for that same evening.

A few minutes later the resolute voice called back. "I've reserved a table at Nettuno, this wonderful little— oh, you know it? Great. I made the reservation under my name, Rega. It's really Regina, but my friends call me Rega. See you at eight."

Rega-Regina turned out to be a small person with a face as resolute as her voice, and a stunning vocabulary to boot. "Okay, so you're the writer, and I'm in charge of script production," she said, when Giuseppe brought us the first espresso. "Anyway, we've got this idea, like a completely new take on Tarzan. Now, we need to make the whole thing a little more mainstream—you know what I mean? We don't see this guy like some outcast from civilization who got lost in the jungle. We're looking at him more like some kind of way to harmonize nature and civilization, body and soul. That's *there* in the subplot, but there's not really enough of it there. Tarzan as a new kind of man, if you know what I mean." Rega reached for a napkin to wipe her glasses, which had fogged up from the hot espresso. I noticed her frames were Yves Saint Laurent.

"So what we're after," she went on, "are scenes and dialogue which will show him up close, so people can feel his pain as well as sense his greatness, and really convincing too. For the past couple years the market's been flooded with all sorts of buffed-up hero types. We've got to steer clear of all that or else we're gonna get blown out of the water. So we're gonna make Tarzan more mainstream, in a nineties kind of way. What we're after is a guy with a kind of . . ."

". . . hardened sensitivity." I finished her sentence. Part of my work involves reading publishers' catalogues, which is where I first encountered this meaninglessly ambivalent expression. Evidently all the media had simultaneously decided to declare the current version of man passé.

"Hardened sensitivity," Rega repeated, and for the first time I saw a smile soften her rigid features. "I'm going to write that down. You can go on and focus that idea in the first plot point." She gave her head a little shake, as if to make certain it was still attached to her neck.

I signaled to Giuseppe, and ordered a glass of grappa. I almost said, "I'll have like a glass of grappa, if you know what I mean."

Wistfully I thought of the people of the Dong, whom I had abandoned for a Tarzan I barely knew and a woman I wasn't sure I wanted to get to know any better. I thought of my "toothless elder" and decided to test one of the sayings I had intended to put in his mouth, making, of course, the necessary changes to fit the context.

"Tarzan is the cliff," I said solemnly, "which must now return to being stone." Actually the image comes from the Japanese national anthem, a wonderful tenth-century poem set to some very unfortunate music. And even though the Japanese anthem had little to do with Tarzan, I noticed I had succeeded in impressing Rega-Regina with a second appropriately incomprehensible remark. I was almost enjoying myself, so why stop? "But tell me, how do you see this man of the future, this creature full of hardened sensitivity?"

My producer once again put her glasses on the table, closed her eyes, and rolled her small head, as if she had been asked to place herself in a trance. "Actually, we're not talking casting just yet," she said after a moment. "That comes later. But I can image him very clearly. This is a man who really knows how to stand up to his fate. He's supple but strong, tough on the outside and soft on the inside, and even though he can be emotional as hell now and then, he doesn't go around screaming his head off like he used to."

"*I* know!" I said. "Let's have this Tarzan of the nineties be steatopygic, with the kind of big round buttocks still found among certain African peoples that serves both as a reserve of fat for hard times and as a cushion for the spinal column. With all that swinging from branch to branch, Tarzan needs something to land on. That's probably why the old Tarzan used to scream so much. We could have a scene where he's practicing kundalini yoga on a thick branch—let's say the famous exercise of the life-snake, which drives all the energy from the loins up to the head. That would be erotic, chiropractic, and at the same time add a certain multicultural medicinal realism, capable of harmonizing European man with the esoteric Far East and exotic Africa. And of course he'd have to keep his trademark loincloth—though it probably shouldn't be made from any endangered species."

"That's terrible," Rega cut me off, "a real ratings killer."

I lit a cigarette and very carefully blew the smoke toward the neighboring table. Without my asking, Giuseppe brought me another glass of grappa: men always sense when their own kind are in need.

"All right," I said, "let's forget about the film for a minute. What kind of man would *you* want?"

"Well, keep this to yourself, but personally I'm all for the old Tarzan," answered Rega-Regina, now very agitated. "If it's one thing I hate it's these limp-dick victims of the women's movement, these weasely wimps always making excuses for themselves." Dark red storm clouds were brewing underneath the gentle rouge on her cheeks. "They're just not enough of a challenge. I want a man who knows when to take charge, who knows when to flex his muscles. I want a man who can move like a cat and fight like a bear, and I don't care if he does scream every now and then or even if he looks a little grungy." She reached out and grabbed her own less-than-grungy glasses, and I waited for the reaction of her cervical vertebrae. This time it came in the form of a jerky little shrug, as if she were shaking off a raven that had been whispering heretical thoughts into her ear.

"Of course that's just my private opinion and doesn't have anything to do with our script, so don't go using it as a guideline. Give me a cigarette, please, would you."

Nettuno is furnished with rustically wide tables, so I had to lean over pretty far to light her cigarette. Ergonomic advisors are right to warn against this kind of bending, which in this instance produced the feared result, the strident protest of the lumbar vertebrae. And while I didn't scream my head off like the old Tarzan, I was certainly not above complaining in a nineties kind of way. Whether I was able to stand up to my fate—or simply stand—was another matter, however, and it would take a very kindly disposed observer indeed to view my reaction as an example of "hardened sensitivity." The ever attentive Giuseppe brought me a glass of water.

"If you ask me," I resumed, after the first flashes of pain had passed, "it's quite likely the man of your dreams will never again exist."

I slid back into my chair, only to release another audible cry of pain.

"Besides," I went on, gritting my teeth, "your old Tarzan could move like a cat and fight like a bear, but all he could say was 'Ungawa!' Maybe there's a connection. In any case, today the whole sex seems threatened with terminal stiffness. Just compare Johnny Weissmuller to Arnold Schwarzenegger. And it's a worldwide phenomenon, too. I've recently completed a thorough investigation of several tribes found in southwest China which proves beyond doubt that there, too, the incidence of male back suffering has increased—to the point where certain traditional rituals can no longer be performed! Spinal stiffness is striking men from all walks of life. And of course in the erotic sphere—"

"You've been talking about yourself the whole time, haven't you?" I could hear the producer's mocking tone despite my heavy breathing. "I should have caught on *ages* ago. Anybody who complains about the same thing more than three times in five minutes is just calling attention to themselves. That's, like, an old psychological rule. And I don't know about your worldwide-epidemic theory. To tell you the truth, it's hard to imagine you were ever the kind of guy who used to go swinging from tree to tree."

The pain and the grappa had put me in a fighting mood: "Actually it's, like, an old physiological rule that it's the truly active individual who ends up paying the most for his physical accomplishments," I countered. "Surely you didn't get that crick in your neck from sitting in a rocker all day doing embroidery—or did you? But getting back to Tarzan, why don't you just go on and make him a woman? He has no future as a man. Once upon a time, modern man was a creator, but now he's the victim of his own victory over nature, as I'm sure you'll find out if you care to consult with any physical therapist."

Rega disdainfully shoved aside the glass of Sambuca which Giuseppe had served her as a courtesy. "I assume we're splitting the bill?" she asked icily.

My piece on the Dong culture in southwestern China was a huge success. Even several scholarly journals made reference to it.

Ninth Vertebra

AN EARLY HUNCH

One of my shortest careers was as a pall-bearer. It began on January 2, 1967, and ended April 21 of that same year. But even in this short span of time I managed to reach the peak of the profession. My meteoric rise is well documented—my picture was in all the papers—but since only a few of my friends know the circumstances, I have decided to tell the story here. Besides, the whole affair provides some insight into the origins of my current stressful situation.

It all began with a misunderstanding: the local draft board had sent notice requesting me to report for duty at some army barracks on a specific day and a specific hour. At the time I was enrolled at the university in Heidelberg, where I was pursuing degrees in Chinese studies and theology, two very exciting subjects which seemed to me far more worthwhile than the "armed service" mentioned in the draft notice. Of course, when I was about twelve or thirteen years old I was crazy about guns, but over the years my passions had changed, and by the time I was drafted I was very devoted to Eastern mysticism. So I dialed the number printed in the letterhead and informed an official that as a practicing Buddhist, I would have to decline their offer to serve in the military.

The voice on the other end replied that a note be made of my stated objection but that a written petition would be required to formally initiate my application for objector status. Besides, even if I ultimately did qualify for an exemption, I was still required to appear at the appointed time for a physical examination.

Anyone familiar with such examinations knows that they are focused only on the candidate's superficial, physical health. The spiritual condition of the future soldier is completely ignored. Back then I was so thin from head to toe that I looked like the Aristotelian definition of a line as the shortest path between two points.

"That will change," proclaimed the jovial examining physician. "Nobody goes out the way they came in"—and his pronouncement proved true in my case.

A few weeks later I was called to appear before the commission whose job it was to determine the validity of my grounds for objecting to serve in the military. Undaunted by their patently foul mood, I explained to the members of the commission that immediately upon receiving my draft notice I had informed the authorities of my religious convictions. One of the grimmer-looking officials, whose name I later learned was Stichnoth, began rummaging through some files. His sharp teeth and claw-like way of clutching the papers suggested an extremely predacious nature.

"Here is the notation," Stichnoth barked. "Let me see . . ." Suddenly he started to grumble with laughter, 'Tilman S. expresses telephonically'—here Stichnoth started laughing so hard he had to interrupt his reading. 'Tilman S. expresses telephonically that he considers every life form worthy of protection because he is a practicing Tourist.'"

The foul mood vanished in a flash. Hands clapped against thighs, glasses came off, tears were wiped from cheeks. Stichnoth was buckled over. "'As a practicing Tourist'"—he went on shouting above the hubbub—"'as a practicing Tourist he cannot wear a uniform. He cannot carry a gun and he cannot fight any Russian, because he is, as he says, a'"— Here Stichnoth stretched himself as high as he could, raised his arms up, and gave the signal for the entrance of the chorus:

"Practicing Tourist," the commission sang out with glee.

Then and there I knew it was a lost cause; after all, I had learned in a seminar on rhetoric that public debates are often decided more by mood than by the content of the argument. So I wasn't surprised when a month later I received a letter informing me that Buddhism did not constitute a valid objection to military service, wherefore my petition for such status could not be granted. I decided to appeal my case. In the meantime, I had no choice but to report for duty.

It was a bleak fall day when I received my uniform. The black collar insignia identified me as a member of an "Attached" company of "Engineers."

The main task of this particular company, as I learned

in the weeks that followed, was to help friendly forces advance and to prevent unfriendly ones from breaking through. In wartime these units are chiefly involved with bridges: they either build them or blow them up, depending on which way the battle is going.

Obviously the army didn't feel this work demanded any special engineering talent or previous training. On the contrary, at the start of what was euphemistically called our basic "education," the sergeant explained to us that all it took to be a good engineer was that he be "stupid, strong, and watertight."

Based on my experience, there's little I would add to this characterization. Up until Christmas we worked on a drill known as "heavy load transport." At times we transported these heavy loads under simulated conditions of "attack"; at other times we were ordered to perform a "strategic retreat." We carried steel carriers and wooden railroad ties, huge cement blocks and bulky pontoons. Most of the time we had to sing, too. It rained a lot that autumn, and I was homesick for my books.

Meanwhile, my body was growing broader and broader. Muscles began to develop in my neck, shoulders, and upper thighs. Now Aristotle would have called me a trapezoid. Shortly before Christmas the quartermaster had to issue me a new uniform jacket.

I almost forgot about my Buddhist objections to military service, for other gods than Buddha reigned in my new surroundings. They wore stars on their stiff epaulets, and their utterances were far from sublime. Nor did they smile benevolently on graduate students.

But I had not been forgotten; after all, this was a democratic state that respected its citizens' religious rights. Of course months had passed in the meantime, and while the wheels of justice were turning I had discovered how to bend my knee a little to shift weight onto the less experienced man behind me. I had learned to hoist and lower heavy objects following barked commands of, "Up!" or "Down!" with the least damage to my skeletal structure, and I even knew all the verses of all of our songs by heart.

Finally, the officials of the democratic state contacted my company commander, who called me into his office. It turned out that my case caused him extra paperwork, so I was subjected to a good deal of heckling, reproaches, and threats. The commander hated everything written, except certain operating instructions for heavy equipment, but even these had to be composed with the utmost brevity so as not to arouse his displeasure. We—and by that I mean the company—had already damaged two transport cranes because the commander refused to read the instructions regarding the use of the mobile arm. And then there was the embarrassing incident during the flood of 1966, when we constructed a bridge twice as long as necessary because . . . believe me, you really don't want to know.

"Have you ever thought about death?" the commander asked me. "You're a graduate student, aren't you?"

I clicked my heels together: "Sir, in the course of my reconnaissance of Buddhist philosophy the theme of death has on occasion indeed been encountered."

"This is obviously not the place for you," the captain

said, and I almost thought I heard a hint of regret. "The fact is, you don't want to dirty your hands by picking up a gun. But since you've already studied death in school, and since we've done such a fine job teaching you to carry things, I'm going to let you transfer to an outfit where both talents will come in handy. Dismissed!"

The Burial Guard was a loose assortment of men pulled from all different branches of the army. It was commanded by a major whose forebears had inscribed their names in the annals of the German military.

Most of the time we were drunk. On cola with rum or cola with whiskey. So I don't really remember how many other Buddhists had been transferred there. I do remember that whenever we were called into action, our chief concern was to make sure the German flag and the symbolic Prussian helmet didn't go rolling off the casket while we were lowering the deceased into his grave. Particularly because our unit was equipped with only one of each.

None of them was as well trained in lifting as I. Whatever the terrain, whatever the wood used for the coffin, I was able and willing to show what I had learned with the Engineers. My comrades followed my example, and whenever he was sober, our major was visibly proud of me.

At first we only handled privates, but soon we were giving noncoms and even a few lieutenants their final send-off. The coffins increased in weight as the deceased increased in rank. In early February we learned we were soon going to be entrusted with captains, and maybe even a colonel or two. Our major was dreaming of a new promotion. In the evening he would often invite me over for a round of drinks, in order to philosophize about what he called "the big connections." His perennial favorite was a proposed memorial tribute he was working on, although he never seemed to get much further than the title: "The Burden of Bismarck."

And then Konrad Adenauer died on the 19th of April.

The news reached us at the conclusion of a small burial at a cemetery in the neighboring village. The major ordered us to assemble and explained, with some emotion, what this death meant for world peace, for the future of the Western alliance, and for the troops that he commanded. Apparently he had already received a confidential tip that the state funeral would be one of unprecedented pomp and ceremony. The major referred to certain official secrets he could not discuss, the dignity of death, and mumbled something about "The Burden of Bismarck." Then he put us all on standby, and even in the confines of the barracks we were strictly forbidden to imbibe intoxicating beverages.

At about ten o'clock that evening he called me into his brightly lit office. The wall behind his desk was covered with military maps on which all possible routes from Adenauer's residence to the Cologne Cathedral were marked in dark red.

"We have to be ready," said the major with a hoarse voice, "ready and, above all, determined. The exact route for the procession has yet to be decided, but the operative units must be prepared for a walking distance of over one hundred kilometers. I have signaled our permanent readiness to the responsible authorities. For the moment, we are holding ourselves in disposition for a mobile intervention. People in higher places have already taken notice of us, and I have no doubt that we will be called in as part of the procession. Grab a glass, the bottle's in the refrigerator. How much does a state coffin like that weigh?"

The question caught me off guard. I muttered something about the type of wood, the metal casing, the weight of the body. The gin bottle was still two-thirds full.

"We'll simply add all that together and multiply by two," declared the major. "There are some old radiators on the parking lot, we'll have them filled with water immediately. In a half hour all the men will report to me. You'll teach them how to carry the things with dignity, I'll polish your drillstep."

Not until early the next morning did the major call a halt to the exercise he had dubbed "Operation Adenauer." Most of my comrades could no longer pull their socks up to regulation height or hold their beer bottles to their lips without help.

The next two days passed in an anxious state of waiting as we progressed from standby to alert. Uniforms were made to sparkle, boots were waxed and polished. The filled radiators were at the ready on the parade ground, but the physical condition of the troops prevented the major from continuing "Operation Adenauer."

"We should consider it a success," he confided in me the next morning, "our first real success, in fact—that we were even under consideration. And by some very top brass, too. I only have one thing to say: The Burden of

Bismarck. I only have one thing to ask: Where were you then? Did you stand with Adenauer?" He laughed knowingly, a little too loudly, and I could smell on his breath a certain relief.

The news that we were no longer in the running spread among the men like wildfire. The incidence of illness skyrocketed. The canteen staff personally delivered the beer to our barracks.

I, myself, was no longer the soberest soldier in the army by the time I saw the major standing before me. Actually, "standing" is not the right verb. He was rocking before me like a boxer who's just endured a hail of blows but won't go down. Little red veins were popping out of his face, reminding me of the map behind his desk. *Replacement!* he cried out. *Hurray!* Then he waved for me to help him steady his balance.

A half-hour later I felt the full measure of his happiness. Of course, if everything went according to plan, we would not personally lay hands on the casket. But we had been commanded to be at the ready. And not on some obscure streetcorner, no; our place was in the center of things. Of course, the longest leg of the procession would be covered by boat ("No spunk in their backs," was the major's dismissive commentary), but we would be right there where the music would be playing.

"Tomorrow morning"—the major placed his arm on my shoulder—"we will be standing inside the cathedral, on both sides of the high altar." The whole affair was beginning to sound more like a wedding than a funeral.

We did indeed have to report to Cologne in the middle of the night. The nave of the cathedral was buzzing with uniformed stand-ins for the VIP mourners. The funeral march-step was being drilled to the sound of muffled drums. Security measures were rehearsed, such as removing possible fainting victims. There was even a duplicate casket, which the supple members of an Honor Guard battalion raised and lowered as effortlessly as if they were rehearsing Stravinsky's *Rite of Spring*.

"Our watch doesn't begin until 0400," said the major, "so we have time for a little more drill."

We left the church, and since we hadn't brought the radiators, we tried to hoist our armored personnel carrier onto our shoulders. Unfortunately the left side of the formation misunderstood my instructions and we teetered into a dangerous diagonal position and were forced to abandon the exercise.

The major cursed us but without much conviction.

Notwithstanding this minor mishap, we managed to take up our positions at the appointed time. We had been called to stand for four hours only, as a reserve watch before the procession arrived. We were scheduled to be relieved at 0800, exactly two hours before the beginning of the solemn requiem, and no one expected any complications.

Apparently we were mistaken. At 0800 there was no relief in sight. Still, standing was one thing we had learned to do. Meanwhile choirs began to rehearse their numbers, the organist checked his volume levels, and somberly-attired security guards combed the church for hidden explosives.

Another hour and still no relief. We stood and waited.

The cathedral began to fill up. Suddenly I spotted Charles de Gaulle, Lyndon B. Johnson, and Heinrich Lübke, all moving toward us, with measured step. And behind them, the casket, gliding in on the shoulders of the chosen—perfect rhythm, perfect posture, perfect bearing.

The cameras of the world press flashed all around, acolytes swung their censers.

Fate was marching toward us, too, toward my comrades and me, as we stood beside the high altar, ready to defend Heinrich Lübke, Charles de Gaulle, or Lyndon B. Johnson, or quickly spirit out the casket if the situation so required. As the dignitaries stopped in their places of honor, Fate marched on into our midst.

At the extreme end of our flank stood a toolmaker from Duisburg, a man who had always struck me as the incarnation of calm. We all admired him for his solemn bearing and his upright posture, which had leant dignity and respect to so many burials. And now this stalwart soldier could no longer control his bladder.

Now he had to pee. And so he did, into his boots, without changing his expression—as we had all been instructed to do in case of emergency.

Later I tried to figure out why, out of all the ceremonies we had attended, it had to happen at that one. Was it because we had been standing for six hours without moving? Or had the man been so humiliated by the perfect performance of the Stravinsky dancers? Looking back, I suppose the conditions in the cathedral were more to blame than anything else. It was, as I said, April, and cold and damp.

Once we caught the first sharp whiff, none of the rest of us could control ourselves any longer.

The then-reigning statesmen have since been carried to their final resting places, so I can't inquire how they felt when that mix of incense and urine first assailed their nostrils.

"Men," said the major, once we reassembled, "I was proud of your bearing."

My mother cried when she saw my photo in the paper.

Tenth Vertebra

PANDEMONIUM

News of the events spread quickly through the city, changing with every telling, and caused quite a stir. To this day no one knows why it took over a week for the authorities to figure out what the hell was going on.

Even *I* failed to appreciate the significance of the first incident, which occurred at the intersection of Maximilianstrasse and the Altstadtring, just where the people driving up to the Governmental Palace cross paths with those anxious to leave it. At exactly nine-thirty-seven in the morning, the traffic light that controls the intersection gave a series of red blinks and then went out. A policeman arrived on a motorcycle a little later to direct the traffic by hand—a strapping hulk of a man with practically no forehead and an abundance of pimples. Later it turned out he also had a speech defect, although that fact had no bearing on the case.

The owner of the Italian restaurant situated right at the scene described to me that same afternoon what he saw happen. Evidently the policeman donned his white gloves, placed his whistle between his teeth, and proceeded to wave the drivers through the crossing, first the north- and southbound cars, and then the east- and west-. The traffic was restored to its usual spurtlike flow—until, all of a sudden, the policeman's arm froze in midair.

What then transpired was, according to the owner of the Italian restaurant, a true *spettacolo*. One collision set off another, creating a chain reaction of unprecedented proportions. Over a dozen government limousines were involved, a fact that actually reassured many onlookers: perhaps now the authorities would at last deal with the growing congestion in the city.

And indeed, within a few hours, various government agencies had transformed this unplanned stoppage of traffic into a systematic chaos. Finally a military helicopter flew in a more flexible policeman and rescued his rigid colleague. The man was hoisted up and away like a monument that had fallen into disfavor. "Just like they did with Mussolini's statue in my home town," said the restaurateur.

The incident itself would have been a good deal less newsworthy had it been an isolated occurrence. But as it turned out, other odd events were taking place elsewhere in the city at the same time.

A near riot broke out in the park next to the old arsenal as a result of an apparent provocation by a certain Werner F. According to the testimony of Jacob S., this Werner F. had approached him and raised his arm in the Hitler salute while he, Jacob S., was simply minding his own business. "As a confirmed Social Democrat I couldn't just take that sitting down," Jacob S. testified before a magistrate. "And when the man ignored my repeated warnings, I had no choice but to defend myself."

Werner F., for his part, claimed that he was just reaching for his hat to hold it out for a little donation, when a violent spasm seized his lower back and rendered him completely immobile. Before he knew it he was being beaten and called a "g——d—— m——f—— Nazi," but he was so stiff he couldn't even defend himself. Werner F. further testified that he had no "real political convictions," although he had long been opposed to "reactionaries and terrorists" of any stripe.

As it happened, however, a number of bystanders rushed to his aid. Whether they fancied themselves protectors of Werner F.'s right to free expression, or whether they were rallying to a cause they had once supported, or whether they simply wanted to break up a noisy fracas, the authorities were unable to determine. By the time an armed antiterrorist brigade had restored order, the nearby hospital had admitted twenty-three people with injuries ranging from superficial to critical. A policeman was rumored to be among the casualties.

Not even the courthouse was immune. In three separate courtrooms, the identical scenario took place: when the bailiffs announced the entrance of the respective judges, each of them female, with the standard "All rise," over half of the parties present refused to budge from their wooden benches—whereby it was noted that the protesters consisted entirely of men. So strong, in fact, was their conviction that plaintiffs and defendants alike joined in the sit-down protest.

"They just sat there like lumps on a log," recalled Verena A., who herself had been arraigned for a moving violation.

The judges responded with repeated warnings which soon escalated to a barrage of threats and ultimately exploded in a rash of fines and prison sentences for contempt of court. But the protesters continued undeterred, so that in the end the judges had to call for the rooms to be cleared "with force." Even this measure, however, failed to restore order, largely because the enforcing arm of the state itself had frozen up, stricken with a lameness that—as was later entered into the protocol—"effectively prohibited the officers from executing their duties as charged."

The Ministry of the Interior hurriedly assembled a crisis staff which included both the Surgeon General Emeritus Professor Dr. Waldemar M., as well as his longstanding enemy, Chief Police Psychologist Dr. Karl-Heinz P.

Naturally the appointed specialists failed to agree on a diagnosis. Professor M. spoke of a "galloping lumbago" unleashed by a hitherto unknown Eastern European virus, while Dr. P. attributed the epidemic to a "mass male hysteria," as described in an early letter of Freud to C. G. Jung. The two experts began hurling insults and incomprehensible ideas back and forth across the room like glittering poison darts.

"But what the hell are we supposed to *do* about it?"

Minister G. demanded to know and brusquely broke off the debate. His disdain for medical experts of any stripe was undoubtedly related to having flunked Latin in high school.

A young advisor pointed out that if the cause really were a virus from Eastern Europe, then the matter properly fell in the jurisdiction of the Department of Foreign Affairs. "Conceivably, it may have some bearing," he continued, "on the revisions underway regarding government policy toward so-called economic refugees."

"This is not a virus!" shouted Dr. P., "this is epidemic hysteria! And we must deploy as many trained psychologists as possible in order to keep it from affecting other parts of the male anatomy!"

But no one was listening to him anymore, and when Professor M. made mocking reference to "presumed psychosomatic symptoms of a mass devirilization," Dr. P. stormed out of the room.

The Chief of Police suggested a general quarantine of the infected, "just as a preventive measure." While this proposition found some support, it was ultimately rejected when the Surgeon General Emeritus pointed to the high risk involved for the officers who would be taking part in the operation.

"It is entirely likely," he explained, "that they would be unable to wield their sticks, not to mention use their handcuffs."

After a moment of silent mulling, the young advisor again piped up: "And what," he asked, "if we mobilize only our female security forces? As far as I know, they are well trained and perfectly reliable. We could call them in immediately. Besides," and here he looked at the minister, "that would demonstrate our commitment to the principle that equal opportunity to serve means equal readiness to sacrifice."

The minister slowly rose from his seat and, smiling, walked around the table to the grinning advisor and slapped him so hard he tumbled out of his chair. Then he bent over to help the poor man up, when, all of a sudden, he too let out a cry of pain.

"I'm sure you've already thought about what the press would do with that," he thundered, clutching his back. "I refuse to be shown up by a bunch of girl scouts! You are an imbecile! An idiot! A flaming feminist! Get out of my sight!"

By now the advisor's cheeks really did look on fire and he ran out of the room as quickly as his lower back would let him. The commission sank into silence. Alarm sirens could be heard through the smoke-tinted windows of the chancellery.

Finally the minister spoke. "A symbol!" he cried out. "We have to come up with a symbol! When there's nothing to be done, at least show some sign that you're doing something. Some sign of resolution, of masculine determination!"

All eyes were fixed on the minister.

"Let us," he declared solemnly, "let us add another traffic signal."

The sirens abated, and suddenly, as if by magic, everything was over.

Eleventh Vertebra

THE MELON

It's amazing that Alejo is still able to walk upright. He lives in a dilapidated stone house plagued by drafts from the constant sea breeze, which the locals call either "salt-sower" or "toad-tongue" in their Spanish dialect, depending on their mood. This wind is constantly licking at their linens and laundry with its wet, salty tongue and causing everything to mildew. And, of course, damp bedding is murder on the back, although perhaps neither Alejo nor his family have read the fascinating scientific literature on the subject.

Alejo's upright gait is all the more amazing when you consider that he is a shepherd, and not on some flat plain or steppe, either. No, the valley where he lives—and where I used to spend my summers—is steep and stony, although that doesn't seem to matter to the sheep. If they slip or slide they just climb back up again and go about their business munching and bleating despite the degree of incline, just as generations before them have done.

For humans, however, it's a different story. Steep terrain is just as hostile to our lower backs as damp bedsheets. The subtle muscle structure designed to enable us to move with ease on smooth terrain is extremely sensitive to the sudden shifting of weight caused by uneven ground.

Some years ago, Alejo inherited a little money and bought an old motorcycle, which can be back-friendly enough if driven on a plush, asphalt-paved street. But the roads on Alejo's island only serve to connect one pothole to another, and when people talk about "streets" they are invariably referring to the district capital. When I expressed my concerns to Alejo he seemed to hear what I was saying. But instead of trading in his bike for an all-terrain vehicle, all he did was buy himself a shiny, upholstered crash helmet.

This is by no means to say that he is completely insensitive to another man's back pain. Last fall, when "Scrunch" decided to pay me one of his surprise visits, Alejo was so concerned for my comfort that he alerted his sister, Isabell, her husband, Montserrat, and their daughter, Maria. All four gathered around my bed. Maria pounded the bedding and fluffed up the pillow. Isabell presented me with a lukewarm leg of lamb rubbed with garlic, and Montserrat cursed the climate and especially the Socialist government in Madrid for creating it.

"*Hombre*," he exclaimed, "these are hard times, which means you have to face your fate and bare your teeth."

Montserrat always says "*hombre*" whenever he sees me,

and I can't say whether it's because he doesn't remember my name or because he thinks that all foreigners particularly appreciate this form of address.

Having thus inspired me, he then ordered me to stand, face the wall, and stretch my arms as if I were about to be nailed to a cross. I was willing to try anything and began carefully lifting myself out of bed. The women, who had been looking on with interest, suddenly turned away demurely as if I were a crucifix and the cloth around my groin were carved so delicately that it might fall off at any moment.

When it comes to strange cures, it's hard to surprise the experienced back sufferer. But even so, most of us have no idea what it's like to be rammed by a minotaur named Montserrat, first in the left hip and then in the right. Perhaps a picador's horse feels something similar when the tortured bull can no longer distinguish between cause and effect. Incidentally, how Montserrat managed to perform this operation without smashing his head against the wall is beyond me.

"Thank you," I said as soon as I could speak, and crawled back between my sheets. I felt every bit as stiff, and even more fragile, than before and was very grateful even for the damp linen, which offered me some refuge from my savior.

The family looked at me pensively.

"He's lying down wrong," Alejo concluded after a while. "The mattress is too soft, and his head should face east. We should lay him down on the table next to the kitchen window."

I was too weak to protest. Maria and Isabell covered the oak tabletop with a wool blanket, and both men grabbed the bedding on either end of me and dragged me like a freshly bagged deer into the kitchen. As prescribed, they heaved me onto the table so that I was facing east: I could see Alejo's sheep grazing and some young men flailing at the almond trees with long metal poles. Maybe Alejo was right after all; the sight of the sheep had a calming effect, and the picture of the cheerful men swinging their shiny poles in the evening sun reminded me vividly and relaxingly of certain physical exertions I would never again have to face.

Before he put on his helmet, Alejo gave me his shepherd's crook. "I'll be back," he promised. "And if it gets any worse I'll take you to see the doctor on my machine."

The idea of a ride on that vehicle provoked a spontaneous spasm across my entire lower back. Pearls of sweat rolled down my cheeks.

"I'm sure it won't be necessary," I answered, my voice weak, "but thanks anyway!"

Montserrat returned the cognac bottle to which he had helped himself back inside the cupboard. "Tomorrow it will all be over," he laughed. "Two knocks from my shoulder should be enough even for your heavy body. So tomorrow we're going to have a real *fiesta*. We're making tripe, fish-liver-and-bird-soup, and all the desserts you can think of. By then you'll be your old self again, and afterwards you'll be so full you couldn't strain yourself if you wanted to. Besides, you have to come—you understand, for me and my family and my friends it's a matter of honor. After all, I'm the one who saved you."

In parting, he said "*hombre*" to me one more time; Isabell rinsed his cognac glass; Maria fluffed up my neck roll. Then a grateful door finally closed shut behind my visitors.

The field of back cures, as I have said, is one vast tundra. It's easy to lose your way, but you soon learn to read the signs. And while an invitation to a celebratory *fiesta* might have escaped the novice; I knew a bad omen when I heard one.

I also recalled all too vividly how another neighbor, an architecturally obsessed Dutchman, had given Montserrat's house his most rave review: "Relentless in its rusticality . . ." And I was sure the hospitality would be relentless, too; the feast was bound to drag on for hours, with guests tightly packed on wooden benches and not a prayer of escape.

I knew then and there I had no choice: I had to change my departure date.

On my way to the airport the next morning I stopped briefly at Montserrat's in order to personally tell him about the unexpected phone call and whatever other lies I might need to convince him I had to leave *pronto*. I even hoped I'd be able to tell him all this through the open window of my car: while my body was less stiff than it had been—either despite or because of the minotaurian cure—I dreaded the idea of having to get out of the driver's seat.

But alas, although the dogs barked and the chickens scattered, the family stayed inside. So I had to make my way up the gently climbing path across the farmyard, skating through the mud and chicken droppings, until I reached the kitchen. Isabell received my news with polite commiseration, only once interrupting her stirring in the gigantic pot to show me a little bird whose emaciated body was swimming in the fat of her ladle. I was visibly choked up as I said farewell.

I was halfway back to the car when a voice boomed out: "*Hombre!*" and Montserrat appeared from out behind his shed carrying a huge watermelon. "A gift for you," he said as he tossed the melon to me in a high lob. I stepped forward, caught the melon, lost my balance, and fell down, slamming my back hard against the peculiar mix of cement, mud, and goose shit Montserrat has designated as a parking place for his guests.

When I came to I was still holding the melon. I was also hearing voices—a very shrill warning, to be exact, which kept repeating inside my head like a broken record: "Any lifting performed with a bent back is liable to in-crease the strain on the spinal column by a factor of ten, any lifting performed with a bent back is liable to increase the strain . . ."

While I was trying to recall where I had read this, Montserrat pulled me back up on my feet. "Thank you," I said, "thank you, I better be going now. The plane is wait-ing." I jumped into my car and sped off.

It took me several kilometers to realize that something special had happened during or after the fall. I had fallen down, Montserrat had helped me up, and then I had jumped into my car. *Jumped!* For several months I hadn't jumped at all, much less holding a thirty-pound water-melon.

By the next gas station I had built up enough courage to test my hypothesis. Sure enough, I didn't look or feel any different than all the other drivers getting in or out of their vehicles. The yellow-green melon sitting on the passenger's seat gave me a little wink.

"A spontaneous remission," said the doctor, "presumably one brought on by a traumatic shock." They all have some kind of excuse.

Twelfth Vertebra

SKI JUMPING

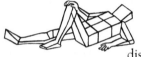 My psychotherapist recommended that I write down the story of my disease.

"Just like you'd write a novel," she said, "except it's one that nobody but you needs to read. Start with your childhood. Anything you can remember having to do with the idea of 'back'—fairy tales, dreams, role models. And most important, write down all your fears, both the ones you've admitted to and the ones you haven't."

"A novel that nobody but me needs to read?" I couldn't hide my skepticism. "How in the world is that supposed to help?"

The doctor raised her eyebrows. "Hmmm . . . ," she said, "a defensive reaction. It isn't very rational, you know, though I imagine it's to be expected. My idea is designed to help you further your self-awareness in the most honest way possible. And to do that, it's best if you're not thinking about how to please your audience."

And then the session was over.

"She wants me to write a novel about myself," I explained later that evening over dinner, "a novel that isn't meant to be published."

"I can't imagine you'd be up for something like that," said Delia, my life's companion, legal spouse (though we have evolved our own definition of spousehood), and mother of my daughter Lena, who now joined her mother in questioning the enterprise.

"You're leaving me out again!" my daughter, Lena, complained. "Why can't you write a book about a little girl who finally loses her baby teeth? Or at least her appendix. And make it funny."

Lena was going through a phase in which the loss of body parts held some peculiar appeal. She also has a stubborn streak, and while I didn't sign on to write her book, I did agree to tell her a story about a great big straw and a camel who lost its hump.

The more Lena listened, the more flourishes I added, so that by the time the camel had regained his hump I realized the doctor was right: I would have to wean myself from the idea of writing for an audience if my "back novel" was going to achieve the desired effect.

So I set about methodically filling index cards with notes and arranging them in chronological order. Before I knew it I was once again in catechism class, learning how to examine my conscience so as to better confess my sins.

The concept of "spinal sin" seemed worth pursuing. I began to sketch out a possible opening sentence: "Every back shall bear the burden of its sins."

"Sounds pretty abstract for a life story," said Delia, peeking over my shoulder. "I thought it was supposed to be about you. I'm going to go watch a little more of the

Olympics." She yawned lightly and gave me a good-night peck on my left ear. "By the way, how are you feeling tonight? Any chance I'll see you later?"

A few years back my wife completed her dissertation on the Pauline epistles to the Corinthians, in which she devoted two chapters to the concept of "*mollitia*"—literally "softness" or "tenderness," but in Paul's usage best translated as "weakening" or even "effeminacy." Perhaps her familiarity with the subject matter accounted for her extreme sensitivity to my plight. Not that she was thinking of me when she wrote those chapters any more than Paul was when he wrote his epistles. Back then, Delia was working as a private tutor, and I myself was regularly participating in crew meets—I can still hear her calling me her "Samson." Even so, it was uncanny how both she and Saint Paul managed to foresee certain problems of mine long before I was even aware they existed.

But how was I supposed to be less abstract? Did she expect me to provide an anatomical account of the changes that affect the spinal processes and their connecting ligaments? Or was I, too, supposed to write about "*mollitia*"? Maybe I should describe the sad metamorphosis from robust man to shuffling homebody, the embarrassment of a grown man asking his wife to tie his shoes, just as he once asked his mother? Or else perhaps I shall dwell on the loneliness of a onetime party animal who now avoids anything that even hints of dancing, or else the envy that springs up whenever the same man sees other fathers toss and twirl their daughters as if they were performing in the Ice Capades?

Of course I could use a bold literary stratagem and portray myself from the perspective of my wife or daughter, full of ironic understanding for the aging patriarch who grumbles each time the weather turns, or for the poor middle-aged fool who can't see what's in the bottom of the refrigerator because he's afraid to bend over.

Trapped in these swirling thoughts, I put pencil to paper and started to draw a snail.

"You know," said Delia, turning off the TV, "I used to be able to watch the men's ski jump for hours. Don't laugh, but there really is something very Zen about it, the return of the eternally constant. A hundred men all poised for death, each one stretched out from head to toe, straight as a ruler, all looking alike in their helmets and glasses. The sad thing is, I can't stand to watch anymore. They still jump the same way—though maybe they hold their legs a little differently. But it's these damned cameras; they use so many angles, it's totally distracting." She lit a cigarette and plopped onto the sofa. "Did you ever do that when you were young? Ski jump, I mean?"

I hesitated before answering. "No, I never had much desire to do that; but maybe that's a good reason to include it in my novel. Dreams and fears, you know, from early childhood on. As well as their later revisions and reworkings."

Delia carelessly let the ash fall to the floor as she always did. "To tell you the truth, it sounds a little trite. Besides, I don't buy it. I recently read that two-thirds of all men with a bad back think of themselves as 'rugged individuals.' Don't tell me a tough guy like you never felt the urge to do something like that at least once."

I knew the study she was quoting: we both used the same haircutter, and his selection of magazines was very limited.

"Maybe I had a secret longing for ski jumping and just didn't want to admit it," I agreed. "You know, a classic case of repression. After all, according to the same study, over two-thirds of the patients questioned confessed they were ashamed to reveal their particular weakness in front of others. And that kind of repression can severely affect one's ability to perform, which in turn can lead to layoffs and all kinds of unheard-of disasters of the economic well-being of the state."

My spouse lit another cigarette before she answered. "When I think about it, I'd just as soon live with a rugged man whose bones ache because he used to be a ski jumper than with a repressed one who suffers because he never was. I mean, from my point of view the one's just as dumb as the other. Anyway, I'm going to bed. See you in the morning." But she just stood there and let another column of ash shatter on the red tiles of my study before adding, "But you've got to admit, it takes balls."

And suddenly everything she was saying became painfully clear to me.

"I don't think," I protested, "that ski jumping really works as a metaphor for sexual drive, even if there is something Zen about the idea of a hundred rigid, helmeted men poised for death all coming crashing down on you. Surely a specialist on *mollitia* like yourself—"

"For God's sake, don't feel hurt because of what I just said, I was just trying to get your creative juices flowing. You looked so helpless there with all that blank paper."

The next time I saw my psychotherapist my writing hand was in a cast.

Thirteenth Vertebra

ARTE POVERA

I met my friend the sculptor Napo more than ten years ago at the Venice Biennale. One evening we happened to be sitting next to each other at a small seafood bar. I no longer remember how we got started talking.

Nor do I recall what language we used, probably a mix of several. But I do remember exactly how he described the fruit crates he had been hauling all day, under great pain, just to earn some money for food and wine. Never before and never since have I seen a fruit crate so vividly recreated; Napo's fingers were so expressive I could taste the apples, the cherries, the honeydew melons.

In the course of the evening I learned that my new friend had been invited to Venice to exhibit one of his works in the Romanian pavilion. The national Artists Guild had arranged for his exit visa and provided a train ticket. Unfortunately, however, in order to exchange Romanian lei for Western currency he needed the permission of a different office.

At that time Romania was a very proud, frightfully poor, and extremely corrupt country. Napo had no connections in the ruling party, and even if he had wanted to, he wouldn't have known whom to bribe. The day of his departure came closer and closer, and still all his petitions went unanswered. Finally he decided to travel to Venice without a lira to his name.

It was his first time abroad, he confessed to me, and the same was true of "his children," the creatures of wood now being readied for display in the Romanian pavilion at the *giardini pubblici*. Most of his children were just about two years old, he explained, using the same vivid gesturing he had used to describe his fruit crates. Apparently there was some connection, but I didn't understand what.

Two days later I ran into him once again at the same place. He had had a bad day, and his fingers were cursing the fruit crates as well as his lack of Western currency.

"Why don't you be my guest?" I asked, thinking I might treat him to a meal.

"You would make me very happy," he answered with a polite bow. He apparently had understood I was talking about a ticket for the Biennale and not a plate of fried sardines. He hadn't earned enough money to pay for a ticket to see his own exhibit.

"I am the father of so many children," he said, "but sadly none of them can feed me."

The next morning we met at the vaporetto and traveled together to the Biennale. We floated past one stop after another in silence, and then, just before we got off at the exhibition, my friend started showing me photographs and talking like a proud father.

"In my homeland," he said—this time his gestures were less vivid since he was holding on to the boatrail—"I am known for making the small the great, for making the Adam whom God made bow down, and all of his descendants who bear their burdens on their back. I am the new carpenter of flawed man." The pictures he showed me were no clearer than his speech; all I could make out were some very blurry objects which could be anything from tiny bodies with dwarfed heads to a messy pile of old warped lumber—with all due respect for modern art. I could find no signs of any backs or burdens, both of which would have interested me greatly, particularly because the relief I had just experienced at the volcanic spa in Abano was beginning to fade.

Napo must have understood my confusion. "Sylvia will explain to you," he said. "I will find Sylvia for you. Sylvia, she is beautiful, she is from my homeland. And all of your languages she knows much better than I. She will be at the exhibit, one hundred percent sure, and especially later tonight—we are going to have a great party. Thank you very much for the ticket."

Then he vanished like a mirage.

My experience with Romanian artists has taught me that their idea of "tonight" doesn't always correspond to my own. The "night" part fits; it's just that they usually mean next Tuesday's "tonight," or next Friday's, or really any tonight other than today's. So I was all the more surprised, and even a little ashamed, when Napo tracked me down that same afternoon at the seafood bar.

"They canceled my exhibit!" he shouted. "But still, we will have our feast, and we will have a manifesto as well.

He spit on the ground and hissed the words "dictatorshit," "resist," and "downfall" as if they were all one syllable. "Here is Sylvia."

He pointed to a young, well-rounded woman with reddish-blond hair who was gracefully powdering her nose in front of an alluring window display of corsets and bodices. Then he kissed me and vanished as quickly as he had that morning.

"I am Sylvia," the reddish blonde was laughing as she held out her hand. "Napo's description of you fits perfectly: he called you 'the shuffling question mark.' But I would have recognized you anyway. Even though I've never met you I feel I know you."

Sylvia spoke German with the melancholy intonation the Germans in Romania have preserved in order to protect themselves against any unwarranted cheerfulness. That same sad inflection formed a charming counterpoint to the humor of her anecdotes.

I soon learned that Napo had quite a history. As a student he had run into serious trouble at the National Art Academy, over an assignment to paint a portrait of Ceausescu. In his painting, Napo gently hinted at the presence of the presidential penis. And this nearly cost him his career, not so much because of the detail itself as because of its size: "small as half a little gherkin," as Sylvia put it.

I also learned that my new friend had renamed himself Napo after Napoleon, which he shortened because the emperor was actually four centimeters taller. "When I knew him, everything was either 'too big' or 'too small,'" laughed Sylvia. "I'm anxious to see what he's up to tonight. It's sure to be a lot of fun."

Sylvia and I finally reached the Romanian pavilion, where we found that the only things on display were three awe-inspiring portraits, one of President Ceausescu taking part in the harvest, and two smaller ones of his wife in the company of some Catholic dignitary.

As for Napo's extended family, they appeared to be hiding underneath a great big, dirty plastic tarp. When I squinted very hard I thought I recognized one or two of the blurry shapes from the photo—perhaps the famous Adam.

"And now," said Sylvia, "I'll let you treat me to an ice cream. We'll have just enough time to make it to the banquet."

The feast took place in Mestre, in the cellar of a long-abandoned church where the only signs of a sacred past were two badly damaged wooden confessionals that had been stacked in a corner. There was no other furniture except for the fruit crates Napo had borrowed from his work. Six of them had been shoved together to create a low buffet, which was bestrewn with sausages, grapes, and slices of cheese. Most guests had brought their own wine. Another crate was placed directly underneath the bare bulb, which was the only light in the room, and which gave everything a matted glow.

Sylvia introduced me to some of her friends. The only names I managed to retain were Ovidiu, Horatius, and Salomon.

Shortly before midnight Napo stepped out in front of

the wooden crate underneath the bulb and shouted a few sentences in Romanian. Sylvia placed herself next to me and translated. "I have a created a golem," Napo was saying, "but he has been placed under wraps by a higher authority."

Horatius put two fingers in his mouth and let out a shrill whistle. "We are *all* under wraps," he said, "your suffering is our suffering."

Napo raised his right hand briefly. "As you know," he went on, "a golem is a creature made by the hand of man, a being who follows the bidding of his master. I have thought long and hard about what a golem should look like."

"Man or woman?" asked the woman next to Ovidiu, cupping her hands around her mouth. "I want to know is it a man or a woman?"

"Climb on your box, we can't understand a word you're saying!" Salomon called out. "Come on, come on, get on the box!"

The audience applauded.

"There is no future for man and his golem," Sylvia translated, then corrected herself—"I'm sorry, I meant 'There is no future for man and his column,' because a column can be bent, a column can be twisted, a column can be wrenched out of its socket or even broken. Therefore what is erect has no future—"

"What about you, how about what's erect with you," interrupted the woman next to Ovidiu, "does that have any future?"

Napo bore the howls of laughter without flinching.

"All of you have at one time experienced the humiliation of being bent, wrenched, or broken. All of you live under a dictatorship."

"Don't get political!" warned Salomon, "they're already waiting for you in Bucharest."

"Let him go on, he's just started!"

Napo raised his hand once more. "I am speaking about a different dictatorship," he continued, "I am speaking about the dictatorship of the vertical. I am calling on you to resist. Western civilization is the glorification of the vertical. From Praxiteles to Brancusi, the history of sculpture is full of examples of the deification of the upright axis. But I say to you, this is a false god, and its worship shall bring disaster. It conjures heroes who never existed, and raises foolish expectations, for no man can ever live up to this ideal, no man will ever show such backbone. Therefore let us renounce it! Let us abolish this tyranny once and for all!"

Here he paused briefly, to let the audience take in what he had said. A young man in a gray felt hat put down his French horn and handed Napo a bottle of wine. The speaker took a quick swallow, wiped his mouth quickly, and again raised his voice: "My second demand is as short as it is radical: the immediate eradication of all pedestals. Because the pedestal, too, is vertical. The pedestal creates nothing but hollow meaning. A work which cannot stand on is own merits does not belong in this world. Therefore, *down with the pedestal!*"

"Bravo," shouted one of the audience, "down with the pedestal!" The applause, at first sporadic, soon swelled to a wave which engulfed the entire room. The man with the felt hat reached for his horn and played a bleating fanfare.

"So what's that you're standing on?" asked the woman next to Ovidiu, after things had quieted down a little. "Isn't that a kind of pedestal?"

"It is a fruit crate," answered Napo, "and if you will be so kind to help me, I will be more than happy to climb down." He really did look uncomfortable, as if he didn't trust himself to get down without help. He crooked his left knee, to hold the weight of his rump, and anxiously tested the edge of his crate.

Ovidiu lifted him up by the waist, set him gently on the ground, and led him to our group. The man with the horn played a dance.

Salomon replenished our wine glasses. "That was fantastic," he congratulated Napo, "amazingly sharp and full of precise innuendos. Except you still have to tell us what this golem of yours looks like, since it's all under wraps at the pavilion."

Napo smiled and pulled a handful of small, cleanly polished pieces of wood out of his left jacket pocket. He placed them on his outstretched hand like a baker arranges crescent rolls before sliding them into the oven.

"Here," he announced proudly, "some leftover knuckles, a few ribs, even a vertebra or two. All I did was saw up fruit crates. I worked the pieces with sandpaper, then I drilled a hole in each one and threaded them together. You can see the result in the photos. My golem is as wide as he is tall, but the most important thing is that his skeleton is like a mobile, always in motion, never out of balance."

Napo passed around the same black-and-white photos I had already seen that morning. But whereas earlier I could see only a blur, Napo's explanation now caused forms to appear which my eyes before had been unable to detect.

"A work of genius," sighed Sylvia. "Napo, without realizing it you have created what the Americans call minimal art."

"He's not a genius, he's a sell-out," declared the woman who had previously been standing next to Ovidiu, "an internationalist sell-out." Obviously the mixture of wines circulating in our cellar had made her a little obstreperous.

"All I did was saw up the fruit crates, rework the pieces with my files, and then sand them with various grades of sandpaper," Napo defended himself. "Besides, what Romanian has the slightest idea of international fashion. I used these old fruit crates because that's all I could find at the market."

Napo started massaging his lower back.

"Now, if you're asking why I don't work in stone like I used to—"

"Fruit crates are the embodiment of *arte povera*," Sylvia cried out, "the idea of trash as medium, as a point of departure, as material to be formed. And since man's spinal column is a piece of trash, it's only fitting that it be portrayed with trash. With splinters of fruit crates and twine . . ."

"Let me tell you how it all began," said Napo, casually smoking a cigarette. "One day, I was in the Carpathians, and I was sawing away at a tall fir tree. All of a sudden I felt . . ."

The horn player began another piece. He played terribly, but I was grateful for the distraction. Men who go on about how their back pain began are absolutely unbearable—it can't be repeated enough. The same holds true for me, although at least my tale featured Adenauer.

Fourteenth Vertebra

PERCUSSIVE MASSAGE

One gray January morning, when the titmice were picking away at their empty feeders and a bout of melancholy had driven me to kneel at my Balans chair, I decided to brighten my mood and treat myself to a "percussive massage," so highly recommended by my medical advisor. The name conjured playfulness and intimacy, and, with some imagination, even a hint of frivolity, which was just what I needed.

It also occurred to me that I would be following in the footsteps of no less a man than Goethe, for the prince of poetry had drummed every one of his *Roman Elegies* on the naked back of his beloved. Not that I envied the poor lady, as anyone who had seen a cast of the writer's mighty hand will readily understand. But the poetic aspect of this image appealed to me, and I was more than willing to recline to a different drummer.

Percussive massage is readily available in my part of

town, since the relatively high median age and income of the inhabitants sustain a number of therapeutic centers. I called the first one listed in the phone book that wasn't obviously part of some national chain.

"Are you quite sure it's not a prolapsed disc?" the receptionist asked twice in her somewhat snooty voice. "Do I understand correctly, then, that you have not experienced any tingling sensation in the upper thigh?" I patiently repeated my doctor's diagnosis, that mine was a case of CLBP, so unfortunately typical for men of "my age," and that the pain emanated from between the fourth and fifth lumbar vertebrae and was by no means due to a prolapsed disc or anything else for which an invasive response seemed called for or even remotely worth considering.

The society of back-pain sufferers adheres to a rigid caste system. Those with a "prolapsed disc" enjoy a higher esteem than those with acute lumbago, who in turn look down upon us "chronics" with evident disdain. In the eyes of the medical profession we are the gray masses, hoi poloi; surgical brilliance would be wasted on us. We present no challenge for scalpel or laser, we provide no prospect of heroic intervention, and thus we offer no motive for medicine to concern itself with our plight. Our banal fate is a longterm metamorphosis into a terminally cartilaginous existence.

"May I ask who referred you?" inquired the snooty voice, after having determined my position in the spinal hierarchy. Nor did she sound any friendlier when I mentioned my doctor, a highly respected physician, and provided her with irrefutable proof of insurance. I was astounded when she scheduled me for the late afternoon.

In all fairness, it should be said that the poor woman was working in acoustically adverse conditions. Over the phone it sounded like I had reached a karate studio by mistake, or else the primate house at the local zoo; the snooty receptionist seemed to be competing with all kinds of grunts and cries, murmurs and yaps, rustling curtains and rutlike trumpetings. And on top of all that a very high-strung orchestra was fiddling away at an evidently painstricken Vivaldi.

As I drove into town I fantasized about relaxing lazily while playful fingers circled on my skin and lyrical rhythms were pounded where my sacrum fuses with the once-mobile part of my spine. Oblivious to the cars honking me out of their way, I slowly shifted from Goethe to Petrarch, from Petrarch to Ovid, until finally I was luxuriating in the Roman baths with the happy contentment of a young child, or an old man.

Obviously this literary daydream was so seductive that it had taken the edge off my usual keenly honed skepticism. Otherwise it's impossible to explain why I so obligingly filled out the forms asking for body weight, marital status, and religion, and why I so blithely proceeded into a huge hall that resembled a field hospital, where many small, numbered stalls were separated by plastic curtains. One of these stalls was mine: I was to undress, I was told. The therapist would join me shortly.

I had been dreaming of fragrant oils, perfumed potions, and pungent essences, of incense offered to the gods of healing—but the priests of this particular temple seemed obsessed with instant pine-needle scent from an aerosol can. Frankly, the brand smelled more of acid rain than sylvan solitude.

Nor did the spiritual atmosphere seem conducive to therapeutic revery, especially to someone like myself, who has always placed the highest value on discretion, despite the current fashion of "sharing intimacies." I consider it a great loss, for instance, that Catholic churches have taken to tolerating a collective admission of sin, instead of insisting on the regular practice of discrete, one-on-one personal confession, regardless of whether the sins committed were venial or mortal.

So when I heard a very loud reprimand for "phy-si-cal sloth and i-dle-ness" coming from behind a curtain two feet away, I cringed. Each syllable was punctuated by the sound of a strong hand slapping against naked flesh. "Physical sloth and idleness," the nagging voice repeated.

"And psy-cho-lo-gi-cal strain." (Here the slapping stopped). "You wouldn't *believe* the people I've seen on this bunk." There followed a list of several prominent locals (here the slapping resumed), with a corresponding account of their physical problems as well as the individual etiologies of each. Some of these people I knew from our local bar; others from TV.

The patient in the neighboring stall mumbled something unintelligible. "You know, I think you're right," affirmed the masseur, and the slapping gave way to the kind of squashy noise a near-empty tube makes when flattened.

"I, personally, see the whole thing holistically," the masseur went on. "What is it you do, anyway, I mean professionally?"

I could only make out the word "programmer."

"I thought so! Completely sedentary!" exclaimed the masseur. "I can see by those love handles. So you're a programmer. Well, when I consider your case holistically, I can tell you that you better think about reprogramming your lifestyle. A profession like that can wreak some pretty severe havoc on the old posture."

To this charge my neighbor reacted with an indignant gurgle.

"Don't cramp up on me now," the masseur interrupted, "you've really got to learn to yield to pressure. But don't worry, I've taken care of cases far worse than yours. The main thing is to keep a grip on yourself mentally. Come on, let's have another go at that weak shoulder."

I heard his shoes clatter on the tile floor, and suddenly the curtain billowed out like a spinnaker. Underneath the hem I caught a glimpse of orthopedic sandals, white socks, and two stripes of tan hairy skin. The right sandal stumbled against the leg of a metal chair.

"Whoa, there goes your shirt," the masseur laughed, "but you don't need it now anyway." The long sleeve of a bright blue shirt spilled into my stall, its starched cuff waving at me like the hand of a drowning man.

By now I was able to read the writing on the wall and

decided to act as quickly as my body would let me. I got dressed and left my stall. At the front desk the telephone was ringing away. Emboldened by my successful escape, I risked two very frivolous passing maneuvers on my drive home.

Fifteenth Vertebra

SPEECH THERAPY

When you consider the mind-boggling complexity of the human body, the countless combinations of bones and muscles and nerves, it's amazing how boring people can be when it comes to talking about their physical problems. And in the competition for the title of Most Monotonous, back sufferers win hands down (and dangling!), as they are more excruciatingly monothematic than even cholesterol fetishists or former nicotine addicts intent on detoxing the rest of the smoking world.

It is my contention, however, that this common obsessive behavioral pattern known as boring conversation is less a symptomatic result than it is a pathological precondition for chronic back pain. I am not a licensed therapist, but if I were ever to find myself on the other side of the couch, I would focus primarily on the patient's anecdotal health. If, for example, someone were to tell me the following story—

"It used to be that the moment I felt my lumbago starting

up, I would ask my wife to jump on my back. That always worked wonderfully. Then she developed a lymph infection in her right knee and we had to emigrate to Africa, where she fell in love with the richest rubber planter in the province, a terrible chess player who ate his hard-boiled eggs with a knife and slurped his soup as if he belonged to some endangered species. So my wife and I split up, and I had to hire a young woman to jump on my back whenever the need arose. She was a Watusi, however, and her head scraped the ceiling of our bungalow, so in the end I . . ."

—I would know that I was dealing with someone whose case was far from critical. To be sure, he may sleep on the same hard mattresses as his comrades-in-pain, he may ingest the same medications, and he may even follow the ski jumping on TV with a certain degree of disgusted yearning, but nevertheless: his soul remains unbowed, as you can see by the energy and color of his narrative.

Sadly, however, such spirited hyperbole is rarely encountered. In most cases of acute lumbar laconism, pain has already gnawed away at the soul to the point of despair, and speech has eroded to nothing more than an occasional grunt or moan. It is then the primary task of the lumbar/speech therapist to help the patient recover his basic sense of articulation.

In practice, the patient must first be relaxed and/or gently prodded into the Active Anecdotal State, in which he proceeds to narrate an actual incident involving some physical crisis. The therapist then shares his diagnosis of both the content of the story and the form of its telling, thus guiding the patient to a fuller understanding of his narrative problem and thereby increasing his chances of cure.

At the same time, the therapist must do everything in his or her power to steer the patient away from statistical findings which only further obscure the patient's sorrows in a series of tables and shaded columns. After all, any treatment that treats every patient as a scared little mouse is bound to inculcate a fear of cats—which, for back sufferers, means spasms, stiffness, and a panicky denial.

Indeed, once the therapist has guided the patient onto the path of verbal recovery, i.e., into the Active Anecdotal State, the therapy would strive to reinforce the uniqueness of each case. A few examples drawn from my own unlicensed practice may serve to better illustrate the technique. The following is by Hans G., a patient well on the way to recovery:

"So I took off the top of my roadster and headed downtown, even though the traffic reporter had announced that there were no more parking places available. Tow trucks were everywhere, garishly flashing their lights. I had to back out of every other street. It was hell. I must have driven more in reverse than I did forward. Still, the idea of giving up never even occurred to me. All of a sudden I felt a sharp pain shoot up my spine, so I simply stopped my car in the middle of the street, holding up the traffic, and stood up in the driver's seat and stretched . . ."

This is an example of a solid therapeutic exposition: clear first-person narrative marked with moments of daring and perseverance in the face of insurmountable difficulties—the suffering *per se* has been pushed into the background. The task of the therapist is to build on the moments of danger and derring-do; they are both elixir and élan for the man who seeks to reupright himself. At the same time, care must be taken to avoid overly simplistic or contrived devices, which can make an anecdote literarily unacceptable as well as therapeutically disastrous, such as ending the above story with the protagonist digressing on his latest X-ray, which in the long run would only undermine his positive sense of self by reinforcing the idea that his problems are less than unique.

The following case of librarian Ernst K. offers a good illustration of how therapy has helped enhance a patient's self-esteem precisely by focusing on the uniqueness of his case. For years this man toiled away, with little recognition and less reward, with the result that both his anecdotal manner and his back suffered from irreversible wear and tear. At the beginning of the therapy his speech was a tedious jumble of incomprehensible erudite jargon, often delivered in a whining mumble. In therapy he learned to focus on his own accomplishments by highlighting the dangers he encountered daily in the course of placing heavy folios onto shelves that were invariably either too high or too low:

"I had no choice but to act on my own. We had suffered a series of cutbacks, call numbers were being issued without rhyme or reason, and I was the only one around who could read Greek. Besides, I had no fear of heights or ladders; after all, I was an avid mountain climber in my younger days. So I

knew what I was up against when I laid hold of a weighty, leather-bound edition of the Septuagint.

Nevertheless, to all of us there comes a time to bid our dreams farewell: only the strong ever attempt to conquer Everest, so only the strong fail in the endeavor. And still—I'd try it again. Anytime. Even under the same conditions!"

Articulation is often the first step on the path to a cure. This is possible even without the support of a therapist, although seldom do such autotherapists succeed in truly polishing their anecdotal style. Let us examine the memoirs of Jonathan B., a famous physician who went on to enjoy a brief political career. His account of his days as chief surgeon is regarded far and wide as being long on wind and short on style, but even so I hold it to be a positive effort at articulation, because it leads him finally to accept his condition. It seems that his own spinal fate came upon him during a routine appendectomy, performed on the son of our local mayor.

"Everything rested on the edge of the scalpel, as I'm always fond of saying. And the man wielding it was no piker, if I may say so, though by his own admission he was a heavy smoker. Still he had a good firm gaze for all that.

"Not so my assistants. Cowards, the lot of them! I could tell by looking at their eyes. Three of them needed disc jobs— that I could tell by looking at their backs. But they waited until I had gone on vacation. Didn't think I could hack it, I guess. I, who personally taught more discs the meaning of fear than any other surgeon in town.

"Even though it was a routine job, I couldn't leave it up to any of those sniveling greenhorns; after all, this was a political

appendectomy, *what with the election coming up and the whole town leaning dangerously toward socialism. A fatal out-come, in the end,* but it couldn't be helped . . ." [my em-phasis]

A literary analysis of these examples will help us derive a model for the therapeutic anecdote. Each story, it turns out, involves a physical crisis. But whereas the onset of the given problem may be seen as the workings of fate, the ultimate outcome of the story hinges on the positive action taken by the sufferer, the acknowledgement of the uniqueness of his particular problem, and the ultimate ac-ceptance of his situation. Wherever this literary scheme is incomplete, the therapeutic result will not be fully achieved.

Now, as I've said, I am by no means a licensed thera-pist, and no insurance company would take me any more seriously than it would a chiropractor. Even so, I feel that my lack of credentials is more than made up for by my enormous clinical experience; after all, I spend several weeks a year at spas all over Europe collecting data from a wide variety of sufferers whom nothing seems to help so much as a properly constructed and delivered anecdote, such as the following, which I humbly acknowledge to be my own:

"Everything began inside our tent, which Hemingway had insisted be left open. He claimed the smell of writers would so arouse the gnu it would lose its senses and even risk attack by mountain lions. I had spent the entire night editing Ernest's last manuscript. As always, exciting passages of superhuman feats were accompanied by totally superfluous, trivial descrip-

tions of ammunition crates, refrigerators, or moth-eaten mosquito netting. While I was attempting to edit this stylistic hodgepodge into a harmonious whole, the wind shifted and started blowing in off the glacier, so that my back . . ."

Ahhh, I feel better already.

Sixteenth Vertebra

VICTIMS OF TRAFFIC

Nobody would call my Uncle H. particularly demonstrative. Perhaps he might seem so when compared to his father—my grandfather—but that gentleman belonged to a generation of men who considered any expression of emotion improper and unmanly.

Taciturn as he may be, however, my uncle left no doubt as to how he felt about the seats in his new Audi Quattro. "Cars these days are just built to look like *other cars*," he said, groaning with reproach, as I helped him into the bucket seat on the passenger side. "In the old days you had to *mount* a car, the way you would a horse, or else step stylishly up into a carriage."

I never once saw my uncle mounted on a horse or riding in a carriage; my own recollections of the old days—in this case, the late fifties and early sixties—have to do with a light-blue Volkswagen, followed by a greenish Opel, which made me nauseous after only a few kilometers. My uncle would frequently have to stop to let me out, and while I tried to regain my composure by the side of the road, he would yell at me: "But I'm sure it can't be the suspension!" All this came back to mind as I seated myself behind the wheel of the Audi.

"The only thing this seat is good for," my uncle continued, clinging to my right thigh with one hand, while the other went searching for the seatbelt, "is to keep you from seeing what condition the road's in. The only reason I can tell what it's like is because my spinal cord feels every little bump. If you ask me, these new things are undignified. Besides, this whole car culture is just one more sign of the creeping decadence!"

I gently reminded him that even though I was driving, the car we were sitting in belonged to him. Following his first attack of muscular rheumatism, shortly after he turned seventy, my uncle decided to heed his doctor's strong recommendation to let members of the family chauffeur him wherever he wanted to go. Of course, the fact that my uncle was willing to relinquish the driver's seat didn't at all mean that he was ready to renounce his title of ownership, or waive his right to choose a new car. Autocratic behavior entwines the male branch of my family tree like thick ivy, and my uncle very much considered himself the man of the house.

His current command as designated passenger was that his nephew drive him all the way to Hamburg to see the Auto Expo, a concept that very successfully hits several male birds with a single well-marketed stone: our appreciation of supple, feline form; our professed hankering for ingenious diversions; our known weakness for technical toys; and our seldom-confessed inclination toward idle chitchat. The impressive variety of cars on display further enables each participant, without challenging his masculinity, to assume any number of roles, so that the male viewers feel free to play macho man in a souped-up hot rod, effete snob in a baby-blue sedan, or environment-conscious intellectual in a battery-powered subcompact.

Unfortunately, as soon as we had finished our first stroll around the exhibition floor, my uncle opted for the role of ardent lover. And as one model after another inflamed his passion, his adrenal glands decided to unleash into his system a large dose of epinephrine, which has the known effect of blocking rational restraint. Like a youthful Don Juan, my uncle moved from one love object to the next, tenderly caressing cables, fondling filters, palpating camshafts.

His doctor had urged him to consider a spine-saving vehicle with "high performance, a high seat, and a high resistance to bad roads and bad weather." My uncle claimed that that was an unequivocal recommendation for a Land Rover—with "more horses than the U.S. Cavalry"—and so we made our way to the British section of the Expo.

By the time we got there my uncle was completely revved up. "You know, what I'd really like is to drive one of these babies standing erect, gripping the reins like a Roman charioteer. Generally speaking, a motor ought to be whipped, from the shoulder, not just coaxed along and jerked to a stop by pushing pedals with your feet." He wasn't joking. This pushing, he maintained, placed undue strain on the lower vertebrae; and besides, the very idea of "disc brakes" only brought to mind some very painful associations with intervertebral ruptures. It was all further evidence of the creeping decadence, and he for one had made up his mind to protest once and for all—"in writing if need be."

"Check this baby out!"—my uncle's use of the term "baby" obviously gave him a feeling of control he had been missing for several years now. He bent deep to inspect the charms of one of the larger masterpieces on display. And then, suddenly, the weight of all his past sins of automotive lust were visited upon him, freezing his back into a stiff arc and leaving him stuck under the silver hood, his left hand welded to a master cylinder and his right waving for help.

When I looked into my uncle's eyes and saw his suffering, I recognized for the first time in my life something akin to a soul. As I was fumbling about to help him out of his precarious position, a young paramedic approached who soon extracted my uncle from the inner workings of the automobile. In his pain, my uncle was unable to express his gratitude: "My brochures!" he yelled in desperation. "Watch out, will you, that nothing happens to any of my brochures!"

The bystanders observed his removal with the respect of hunters who have lined up to bid farewell to a fallen brother. And while no horns were blown, an oppressive, tense silence, such as often announces the presence of danger, set in and lasted for a considerable time. For their part, the vehicles just stood there, motionless, unmasked on their revolving platforms, garishly naked, even obscene. One had already claimed a victim.

The entire group of auto enthusiasts then underwent a sociosomatic change which might be best described as a general realignment. Suddenly they began to behave like aristocratic courtiers: their once boorish movements grew more refined; gruff, grunting commentaries gave way to elaborate displays of eloquence; what had been a slovenly, slouching crowd now became a veritable school of proper posture and elegant bows.

The men rocked gently back and forth on the balls of their feet, gracefully extending their necks. They shifted their weight according to all the rules of ergonomic etiquette before gingerly letting themselves down into one of the automobiles on exhibit. Many a man even relinquished his place in line, contenting himself with a mere cursory glance, as he courteously held the door open for the next viewer, all the while smiling politely, either out of masculine camaraderie or sheer embarrassment.

After receiving the standard injection of novocaine my uncle soon bounced back, in the best of moods. "He who is made to bear the burden of decadent technology is entitled to reap its benefits," he declared, waving a packet of pills he had received at the emergency station.

"Listen," my uncle declared, dragging me over to the Italian display, "those British cars are all too fusty. Let's try out the Alfa Romeos. Take a look at that baby."

I was dumbstruck.

"Don't look at me like that," he went on. "Come on, we don't have all day."

All the way home he was raving about the cobblestone streets of his childhood.

Seventeenth Vertebra

OTHER PEOPLE'S PROBLEMS

Laura and I first met in front of the hotel, each of us politely waiting for the other to enter the revolving door. Our gestures were limited to a smile and a nod, as we were both carrying packages for mailing. Laura's load consisted of two thin boxes which might have contained anything from very flat hats to Linzer tortes or else the literary remains of some poor writer. They were carefully tied with string in the old-fashioned way, so that the name and address of the recipient lay in one little quadrant and the return address lay in another, as if keeping a respectful distance.

I noted these details less because of an immediate fascination with Laura but rather because I was trying to decide whether or not to gallantly offer to take her packages. In the end my fear of literary remains won out; yet when the concierge failed us—he didn't have enough stamps on hand—Laura turned to me and asked if I might show her the way to the post office. She explained that it was her first time in the city. Her voice was husky, with just a hint of a foreign accent. I didn't hesitate a second in obliging her request, and so we set off.

That morning I had woken up with more than the usual groans and grievances, and although my gait can rarely ever be described as vigorous or bounding, on that day the best I could manage was a humiliating shuffle. Once we even had to turn back in the middle of the street, all because the insidious signal jumped to red before we had reached the median.

I say "we," though I was the only one experiencing any difficulty. Still, Laura stuck with me like a shadow. She obviously considered the misshapen figure hobbling beside her part of the larger riddle posed by the foreign city, a riddle for which she would sooner or later find an answer, just as she would for the sooty façades of the houses, the ubiquitous aroma of split-pea soup, and the green monotony of the municipal landscaping.

In the long line at the postal office I learned her profession as well as her name. She came from Krakow, was a conservator of contemporary sculpture, and her flat packages contained some sketches she was mailing to her employer, a gallery owner in Cologne.

This particular post office, as I had discovered on an earlier visit, attracts a clientele highly inclined to protest the rising prices of stamps, very finicky in choosing commemorative issues, and extremely fastidious when it comes to getting—and checking—their receipts. As if that weren't a big enough waste of time, any given clerk may declare an official break at any given moment by hanging out a cardboard sign saying "Temporarily Closed," thereby scattering the entire line and sending the patrons racing to other windows. I normally have little patience for such wilful rudeness, but Laura smiled away my disgruntlement by recalling her "socialist background," which had taught her to cope with every conceivable form of line, from the clearly angled zigzag to the snakelike wave.

Snakes, as it turned out, were very much on her mind, since her current commission involved the restoration of a valuable piece constructed entirely of unopened yoghurt cartons titled *The Serpent Walks Erect.* The owner was threatening to sue the dealer because the serpent in question had reverted to an earlier evolutionary state and could no longer stand without the help of a small scaffold, which distorted the original form of the piece. "Imagine," laughed Laura, "the artist is a vegan. He knows nothing about dairy products! He didn't realize that yoghurt is bound to get all lumped up sooner or later. If you ask me, it's a medium better suited to expressing transience, or even mortality, but not a serpent walking erect."

While she successfully navigated her way through this complicated grammar, she held her packages by the string, one in each hand, and carefully lowered and raised them several times as if that were part of her usual upperbody workout.

She talked with such enthusiasm that I could only listen to her, enraptured. I myself felt as if I had regressed to some larval state of immobility, or else advanced in age like a carton of yoghurt to the point where I, too, was "all lumped up."

Even so, for a lump of larval yoghurt I was not immune to Laura's restorative charms. And my interest was further whetted later that afternoon when I observed her from a telephone booth in the lobby of our hotel. Presumably studies have been made which prove that just as every disease has its secondary symptoms, so every category of sufferers has its own definition of seductive. To me, peering through the tinted glass of the phone booth, Laura appeared the embodiment of all the erotic fantasies a back sufferer could possibly imagine, as she reclined so lithe and lissome on one of the fake rococo sofas that adorned the hotel lobby.

That she appeared to be squandering her magnificence on a young man whom I could see was nothing more than a dimwitted dolt, filled me with a mixture of envy, longing, and hate. Not that anything had happened between Laura and me to offer the slightest justification for this feeling; for all I knew the bodybuilder sitting so coolly in his Armani jacket and crossing his well-pumped legs as if that were the most natural thing in the world was merely her yoghurt supplier. Still, it was clear that some unspoken connection, some powerful drama, was taking place between the two.

Perhaps that's why I was limping so histrionically when I emerged from my phone booth. My back looked like some evil enemy had dipped it in concrete, and I was gasping for breath. Laura spotted me and waved me over. The young man rose casually at my approach.

"Wonderful," he was saying to her, "so we'll talk later." He bent down beside his chair and lifted a massive ancient bronze statue of Buddha off the floor as if it were a little doll made of papier-mâché.

"I'd like to have his problems," sighed Laura, after the

young man went bounding away. She shook a cigarette out of its packet. "The only corrosion he has is on the surface. All he needs is a weak solution of ammonia, a cloth rag, and a pair of rubber gloves. Would you happen to have a light?"

My inattentiveness was only excused by the fact that the word "corrosion" had me thinking not so much of Buddha but of my own back. Happily I found a match, and even managed to bow a tiny bit in her direction as I struck it. So, this young man was more interested in Laura as art restorer than as work of art. In a visible show of emotional release I bravely shifted my weight from one foot to the other.

"Everything I get involved with," Laura went on, with a tinge of bitterness, "is crumbling or shrinking, or else it's dried out or eaten by mildew, but I suppose that's the price I pay for living in the present."

This time there could be no doubt; apart from the mildew, it all fit too perfectly. I was stung to the quick. That's just the way it is; we back sufferers are hypersensitive. I spent the rest of the afternoon recuperating from my rejection, relying on the hotel bar to provide the proper physical, chemical, and psychological support. The half-standing, half-sitting position is particularly soothing for men with my affliction. Once, as I was brooding over my fate, I caught a glimpse of myself in the mirror behind the bar, standing among the beautiful bottles in all my former upright glory.

Eighteenth Vertebra

THE ARC OF HYSTERIA

Closing the curtains to my study always opens my mind; the wide view from my window is so beautiful it distracts me from my work. The trees and the fields and the crook of the river spill over the stringent lines of my arguments like wild splotches of paint. What would have been a sound conclusion, an incontrovertible proof or a clear refutation begins to waver or wriggle or flutter away, and it takes me a long time to dispel the colorful images from my brain.

So when the conversation with Julius turned to the erotic, I drew the heavy curtains shut. My friend is an expert on many things, from Greek art to alpine flora, and a keen observer of detail. He's also an avid debater, and tends to get carried away with his own arguments. And he seldom begins a conversation without some hidden agenda.

So naturally I was a little guarded, if not downright uncomfortable, when the conversation began to focus on me. Surely Julius had not failed to note that my own erotic life had been a little stunted of late, and I was in no mood for him to place me on the psychoanalytic rack.

"Of course," he said, as I poured us each a glass of wine, "the question of erotic desire is not purely physiological. You with your bad back should understand that better than anyone. Actually the very word 'intercourse' smacks too much of commerce and traffic for my taste. The physical act of love is primarily an acting out of psychological fantasy—"

There he goes, I thought. His penchant for analytic jargon was the result of two separate affairs with practicing psychoanalysts. I decided to head him off.

"I know, I know, it's all transference," I said, taking the professional psychospeak right out of his mouth. "Actually the very word smacks too much of banking and real estate for my taste. Besides, what difference does it make what you call it?"

Undoubtedly this was my defensive jealously speaking, since I've never in my life slept with a psychoanalyst, or even just a plain psychologist. To tell the truth, I'd have much too much angst to do so, just as I'd be afraid to invite an interior designer into my apartment or take my mechanic for a spin in the dilapidated Audi I got from my uncle. Call it embarrassment, or respect for privacy, but there are simply some areas where I draw the line.

"Aha! You're resisting," said Julius, reading my body language like a Freudian textbook, "and resisting is a sure sign of repression, and repression is what's causing your block. And I don't mean just with your writing."

I refilled my glass.

"It's incredibly obvious," he went on. "Look"—and here he went over to a sculpture I had just acquired, a female figure with head flung far back, her long curls dangling, her arms outstretched, and her legs snuggled tightly together. This fantasy in bronze and ivory was a copy of a statuette by Ferdinand Preiss, who had given it the uninspiring title *Spring's Awakening*.

Julius gently ran his fingers along the woman's back. "What do you feel when you slowly glide your hand right here, along this exquisite arch?" my friend asked provocatively.

"Envy," I answered without hesitation, "first the concrete envy of the owner of the original sculpture, then the more abstract envy of his limber model. You couldn't get me to hold a position like that longer than twenty seconds, no matter how much you paid me."

Julius sighed. "Try to put it in a larger context."

A shiver ran down my stricken spine. This habit of viewing life as a grand scheme reminded me of college seminars in which the subtlest nuances of a poem or novel were crammed into some crude scheme or structure. Personally, if I want to reacquaint myself with French society before the turn of the century I read Maupassant rather than plow through stacks of statistical findings; I find early Engels more palatable than late Marx; and I always prefer Dante to the professional demonologists of the early church whenever I require an eyewitness account of hell.

"Look at the arch of her back!" my friend bulldozed ahead. "Look at the expression on her face!"

My only response was a blank stare, and Julius decided

to offer me a hint. "I have one word for you," he said. "Hysteria."

I knew immediately he was referring to an essay we had argued over years before, in which a clever cultural historian analyzed Jugendstil poetry, painting, and medicine as a *Gesamtkunstwerk* of the hysterical mind. I myself had always interpreted all those nubile Viennese maenads, with their outstretched bodies and wide-flung arms, as symbols of female submissiveness, but Julius called my attention to their necks, whose stiffness he explained as "a classical symptom of clinical hysteria in its precathartic state." To buttress his theory he referred to Paul Régnard's beautiful photographs of a certain "Augustine," who, just like a ballet instructor, had demonstrated for students at the Salpêtrière hospital the perfectly arched spine of the hysteric. I had responded by pointing out that the same photos, if placed against a different background, could just as easily show a female figure skater performing the famous "death spiral," though without a partner.

I no longer remember who won that particular debate. Probably no one, since Julius knows absolutely nothing about figure skating, and I'm usually so eager to agree— unfortunately—that I don't work out my own opinion until long after the conversation has concluded.

But this time I was determined to resist. "I get it," I responded as sarcastically as possible. "You're saying the male back patient of the 1990s is simply the psychosomatic reincarnation of the hysterical female of a hundred years ago, right? Well, I guess if you ignore the fact that *she* arched her back backward, whereas we tend to bend ours forward . . . ah, but then maybe that difference is simply just another type of transference."

"What can I say?" answered Julius smugly. "Certain diseases are slaves to fashion. They appear, they disappear. But that's not what I'm getting at. We were talking about sexual blocks, were we not? I'm sure you realize that every time you suffer one of your so-called attacks, you curl up in the fetal position. I'm also sure that as soon as you stop being so defensive, you'll realize that there's something deep inside you telling you to hang on to your balls. And the sooner you realize that, the sooner you'll get over this little block."

"Listen, I was doing that long before I even knew what an orthopedist was," I snapped back, realizing I had just lost another debate.

Nineteenth Vertebra

THE KOWTOW

It took me a long time to forgive my friend Pauline Wu for inviting me to her parents' for the midautumn Festival of the Moon. Although there's no doubt that the experience was culturally enlightening, for my back it was cataclysmic. Of course this wasn't due to any evil intent on the part of Pauline; she is much too morally upright for that, and even if, sometime in her childhood, a shadow of naughtiness might have momentarily darkened her soul, the missionaries who raised her would undoubtedly have driven it hence. Surely a Chinese child named after the Apostle Paul could never harbor any deep-seated malice.

I should add that Pauline Wu is extremely beautiful. Chinese poets would have invoked almonds and tender peaches to describe her countenance, shimmering black silk to describe her hair, a dragonfly for her waist, and supple bamboo for her wonderful poise and posture.

Perhaps I should also add that Festival of the Moon today seldom lives up to its silvery-sounding name. More often than not it consists of an ostentatious display of giv-ing, receiving, and devouring moon cakes, which are filled with a cloyingly sweet paste that swells up in the mouth like a puffer fish. It's a miracle the entire popula-tion doesn't simply explode every autumn.

And perhaps I should describe Pauline's parents as well as their house. To begin with, I have never once laid eyes on her mother. Her father, on the other hand, I know quite well, and can state for certain that his appearance would hardly have inspired any poet anywhere to invoke images of fruit or shrubbery or even insects, although a caricaturist might have enjoyed comparing him to some antediluvian crustacean and portrayed his bulging eyes with particularly vicious strokes of the pen. "Old Wu" viewed the world—which was daily becoming more for-eign to him—like a soldier ready to defend the old order at any cost, ruthlessly, defiantly, mistrustfully, megaloma-niacally.

As for their home, it lay in a southern suburb of Taipei, where many traditional houses may still be found intact: its stuccoed walls were dirty gray; its doors short and nar-row; its lamps hung dangerously low. A Central European of average height had to keep constantly hunched over, and even Pauline was always bowing her pretty head. Of course she had done so since she was a child, for this gra-cious gesture is how a Chinese girl shows the respect due to her worthy progenitor.

In the entranceway, we each gave her father the oblig-atory bows and presented the moon cakes we had brought, which he accepted with a laconic grunt before tossing them on top of the dozens of others. Then Pauline dragged me into a dark corner of the guest hall, where we sat down on two cold porcelain footstools. "He's still in a bad mood because of you know what," she whispered, and quickly backed away.

"You know what" had happened a week before. We had missed the last bus; the moon was shining then, too, although not as festively as today; the night air was filled with the scents of unknown flowers, and Pauline had cozily hooked her arm in mine as we turned onto her street.

Evidently I was so enraptured it took me a while to react when four young men suddenly jumped the low wall which separates the Wu garden from the street. I have only a vague recollection of white undergarments and sweaty torsos glowing in the moonlight. But I remember very clearly the long clubs they were brandishing like baseball bats.

"May your way be straight and smooth," I cried out in panic—that idiotic sentence from the grammar book was the only Chinese I could think of. Then I put my arm protectively around Pauline.

"My brothers!" she whispered. "We're done for!"

The biggest of them looked me over and lowered his club. "It's just her German teacher," he said, audibly disappointed, "the fat guy who can't walk straight." In a moment he turned on his sister: "We thought you'd been kidnapped, or even worse. We hadn't heard from you for hours, and Father ordered us to fan out and search the area."

Speak of the devil. Just then Old Wu came out of the door and marched right up to me. His eyes looked as if they were about to pop out of his head; the red veins were even more swollen than usual. It was then I realized I still had my arm around his daughter, and what's more, I had accidentally tugged the slit of her silk dress in such a way that her left leg was bare to her upper thigh. If the old man had been a connoisseur of Latin dance, he might have taken us for a couple ready to tango.

But, alas, Old Wu was not a connoisseur of anything that wasn't Chinese, and I could tell by looking at him that I had become the embodiment of everything foreign and detestable the world over. A hellish curse came foaming out of his mouth and landed as a ball of spit on the dusty ground right in front of the tips of my shoes. Then he spun around and marched back into the house without saying a word.

"It's probably better if I go now," said Pauline, releasing herself from my embrace and fixing her dress.

Her brothers followed her, swishing their clubs through the night air, which no longer seemed quite so sweetly perfumed. Then they started playing at being master swordsmen from the ancient cloister of Shaolin.

Pauline never told me what else happened that evening, but the next morning she asked to have her German lesson moved from late afternoon to early morning, with the sole explanation it was "because of you know what."

And the same "you know what" was exactly why we were celebrating the Festival of the Moon on two cold porcelain footstools in the corner of the hall. Naturally I had brought three times as many cakes as the ritual required and even wrapped them in special paper that was almost impossible to come by anywhere. And as I was traipsing all over town I kept thinking of the Chinese proverb: "A troubled heaven never clears without a storm."

While I sat there wondering who had penned that bit of wisdom, Pauline's brothers stepped into the hall. Each hit his fist against his chest, then bowed ceremoniously before his father and presented the obligatory cakes. Afterwards they retreated into the corner furthest removed from us, and once again began enacting ancient battles.

I confess that I watched them with a certain envy. As a child I had been taught to bow properly; later on, a thin-lipped gymnastics coach had instructed me in how to perform all manner of bends, rolls, and bridges, and finally the army had subjected me to drills such as "carrying heavy sacks," "pinch-ass marching," and "solemn parade step"—all, without exception, utterly unnecessary. My point is that I had had the benefit of abundant physical education, yet what Pauline's brothers did with no instruction whatsoever was far more challenging than anything I had ever achieved anywhere.

Meanwhile Pauline kept staring at the stone floor, as if she expected it to grant her absolution. She didn't see me sneak off to watch her brothers. I don't remember what drove me to do that, whether it was an unconscious attempt at reconciliation or whether I was just the rabbit falling under the spell of the snake. Then again, it's perfectly possible I simply felt bored.

At first none of them noticed me. The three younger ones were all occupied with walking around the eldest in a kind of duck waddle; the eldest was gripping an imaginary staff and periodically thrusting it up through the ceiling. As he did so he would hiss out some command that I eventually understood to mean "Palm tree shoots the moon." Later I discovered that this was a cultural tradition, and every move of the arm, every twist of the rump, and every bend of the knees is accompanied by a melodic response, a saying of veiled obscene content such as "Crane king pecks his great big egg," or "Limp thunderstick, again rise strong."

"Ah-*hu*!" the oldest brother suddenly shouted and aimed his imaginary stick at me. The others broke out of their waddle and pointed threatening fingers at me as well. The floor of the hall began to wobble gently. Somewhere in the shadows a vase broke, sounding a quiet, almost mute lament.

I attempted a slight bow and went back to Pauline, who was still counting the dust specks on the floor.

"Hold your neck like a bamboo reed," she said, without looking up. She spoke with cool detachment, as if she were reading from a medical text.

I sat down and thought deep and hard. Chinese philosophy, I mused, has two faces: the teachings of Confucius and the teachings of Lao-tzu. It follows that Chinese posture has two faces as well: the stiff, pointed finger and the flexible neck. Strict obedience and flexible adaptability. Hard spine and elastic disc. Perhaps this wise balance is the key.

I decided to put my theory to the test, and slowly began to bend, keeping my neck like a bamboo reed, my arm outstretched and my index finger pointed. Then, through a series of carefully executed pelvic tilts, I tried to determine whether the pain that had struck that morning between the fourth and fifth lumbar vertebrae might be fading.

Three or four bends were enough to refute that theory. In fact, I obtained quite the opposite result: my muscles fused together into a ring of steel that throbbed with pain every time I inhaled. I closed my eyes . . .

By the time I opened them the scene had changed dramatically. An extended family, spanning three generations, had entered the hall. Judging by their appearance and dress they came from a remote village.

"Father's tenants," whispered Pauline, looking up briefly.

The tenant farmers had brought presents of their own, which they humbly placed beside the door, as if they feared to contaminate the other packages. The grandfather-farmer barked a command, and the entire family threw itself on its knee.

"Not necessary," muttered Old Wu, but for the first time ever he seemed relaxed, almost cheerful.

The family paid no attention to his mutter. As the ceremony of the kowtow prescribes, they snapped their foreheads three times against the floor, then stood up briefly and began the whole exercise all over.

Toward the end of the second round, Old Wu stood up and grabbed the grandfather by the right shoulder. "I said it's not necessary. Stand up, please, and you others too!"

The sons and grandsons continued politely until the

grandparents had risen, then they sprang up and discreetly brushed the dust from their clothes. "Our most humble wishes for the Moon Festival!" they cried.

Pauline inclined her head my way, and in her deep, dark eyes I read my fate. "It's a very traditional custom," she whispered, "perhaps even reactionary. But did you see how much my father liked the show of respect?" She hesitated a moment, but I could sense what her next words were going to be; it was as if they were drawn in beautiful characters across her smooth forehead. And sure enough: "It's only because of you know what. Afterwards you'll feel a lot better. You know: A troubled heaven never clears without a storm."

"Protest" is too inadequate a word to describe how my body reacted to that. My bones grated, my discs began to howl, and the steel ring of freshly cramped muscle started to sound an alarming gong. "Don't do it!" cried a chorus of all the therapists—physical and psychological—I have ever consulted. "Resist!"

In vain, of course. A man must follow his fate, even if he has to shuffle. May your way be straight and smooth, I told myself. Then, as the ritual commanded, I threw myself down before Old Wu.

The pain flashed in colors I never knew existed; I saw icy blue turn to fiery yellow, then a strident green gave way to a deep pitch-black brimming with misfortune. I tried to detach myself by reciting wise Eastern proverbs. I evoked the supple bamboo and the gentle water that is said to soften the hard stone. I even thought of the Pope, who at that very moment was undoubtedly kissing the tarmac in some unknown corner of the world. Nothing helped. Finally I cursed everyone and everything east of the Suez Canal, and the midautumn moon most of all.

Pauline's assurance that I would feel a lot better afterwards sounded like malicious mockery but for one thing: her father really did enjoy the performance. However, whereas with his tenants he had intervened after the second knee-drop, he permitted me to go on kowtowing to the bitter end. Not until I could no longer move did he deign to stroke me with his staff, conveying, ostensibly, his blessing upon my shoulders.

Pauline's brothers had to carry me out. The two oldest supported me as we shuffled back to where I was staying. The other two sang and pranced and gamboled the entire way.

Twentieth Vertebra

PARSIFAL

The weather was a mix of wet snow and icy drizzle. An oozy slush had covered the dirty gray sidewalk, so that every step was swallowed by a watery squish. There were throngs of pedestrians everywhere. It was Fasching—carnival time in Munich.

At first glance, my friend Michael H., chief dramaturg of the Munich Opera, seemed to be one of the costumed merrymakers. He was wearing a large black greatcoat, slick from the rain; a white neckpiece poking out of his coat made him look like a Biedermeier burgher or a nineteenth-century Protestant pastor. It also imparted a posture Erich von Stroheim would have envied.

Together we might have been taken for a pair of indefatigable carousers: after all, the untrained eye can scarcely distinguish between a drunken swagger and the strategic maneuvers designed to protect the spinal column while negotiating over uneven terrain. Needless to say our particular form of locomotion belonged to the latter category.

Michael H. was wearing this white ruff—which covered most of his upper torso—as the result of an incident he had referred to over the phone as a "burlesque"; he promised to fill me in later on all the gruesome details.

By this point I don't think I need to elaborate on my own physical impediment. At most, I'd like to point out that it's very rare for a CLBP man like myself to form a genuine male bond with a man whose problems are chiefly cervical. The aching back is inclined to view the pain in the neck as a symptom of near-hysterical hypersensitivity. Statistics show that women are the favored victims of this higher form of spinal injury, whereas man in his suffering is best understood from a lower perspective. But since Michael H. had previously seen eye to eye with me on the pros and cons of intensive abdominal muscle training, I knew our friendship could overcome this potential barrier.

My friend was just about to launch into the aforementioned gruesome details when we passed the display window of an orthopedic equipment supplier. In deference to the reigning carnival atmosphere, all the articles on display had been decorated with a kind of lighthearted folly: electrical nerve stimulators were floating on heaps of bright yellow confetti; electric blankets and thermal sleeping bags were ringed with gaudy paper streamers; three wheelchairs were rearranged for an impromptu kaffeeklatsch, their armrests sprinkled with colored powders and festooned with blue and violet balloons that danced in the breeze of a discreetly hidden oscillating fan. A metal walker sporting a dunce cap and two papier-mâché noses was enough to make my friend gasp, and when he laid eyes on a mannikin dressed as Harlequin perched on the Back Saver Automatic Bath Lift, he took me in his bony grip and pulled me away.

"*Nimm mir mein Erbe, schliesse die Wunde*"—"Take my inheritance, close the wound"—wheezed Michael H., and for a moment I couldn't tell whether he was talking about the display window, his cervical ganglion, the recent "burlesque," or the recent production of Wagner's *Parsifal*, which had been mysteriously postponed.

"*Du Allerbarmer, ach! Erbarmen!*"—"All-merciful one, have mercy!" I answered carefully. In school we had had to learn the first act from that opera by heart.

Michael H. looked at me surprised and asked me if I would kindly hail a taxi. Then he invited me to his place, where he promised to tell me everything over a glass of Aloxe Corton, which he had recently come to appreciate as the only effective therapy. Remembering that his spacious apartment was located on the ground floor, I happily accepted his invitation.

"It all began eight weeks ago," my friend explained. "I don't care to name names, but as you know we were rehearsing *Parsifal*. The director had worked out an elaborate production concept he called "The Weakness of the Strong Man." Naturally the idea of redemption was there too. After all, you can't ignore the text completely, but for this director the leitmotiv was to be castration, you understand."

Experience had taught me to nod obediently whenever a theater professional explains some obscure concept and then attempts to make his audience an accomplice to his ideas by tacking on a "you understand." So I nodded, all the while watching admiringly as my friend raised his wineglass. Some years ago a Japanese engineer had shown me a robotic arm attaching finished car roofs in an automobile assembly line: my friend was now executing a comparable sequence of movements, and, just like the robot, punctuated each one with a sharp gasp.

"Amfortas's wound"—Michael H. resumed his narration after the robotic arm had successfully returned the glass to the table—"could, in theory, be located anywhere on the body. There are no unequivocal directions in the script. Conventional directors, especially when they're working in New York, invariably choose the place where Christ was wounded by the Roman soldier's spear. For the singer, that has the advantage that he can simultaneously 'play' the wound and catch his breath. However, according to our conception, Amfortas's wound was in the groin."

I again nodded and added, like an eager pupil: "All in keeping with the leitmotiv of castration. I understand."

The dramaturg wanted to reward me with a nod of his own, but his collar quickly made him think better of it, and he simply gave me an appreciative glance.

"Our costumer designed an outfit that accentuated, shall we say, the groin by means of a brownish-red pigment, thus giving a visual locus to the pain. All of which was fine, except we had overlooked one very crucial detail. . . ."

After an awkward pause, Michael H. tapped the pocket of his coat. I handed him a cigarette.

"A mistake that only beginners would make," he said, after I placed a lit match beneath the cigarette he was holding high in the air. "Everybody in the business knows that baritones have even less imagination than tenors. Once they've been taught to play a wound, then they do so with a vengeance, regardless of where this wound might be. On top of that, no one, including his agent, had told us that our Amfortas had undergone disc surgery two years ago. And we had built a stage with a very steep rake, so that instead of the usual grabbing at his side, he was going to have to double over at every entrance. We should have foreseen what might happen. But it all turned out even worse."

I noticed that the Aloxe Corton was beginning to look more and more like blood, and that I was becoming more and more aware of the mystical connections between male suffering, color symbolism, and intoxication. I would have gladly shared my insights with my friend, but the dramaturg was impatient to get to the denouement.

"Our Parsifal—and I'm sure you know who I'm talking about—is well known for being a very ambitious singer and an irrepressible ladies' man. In his youth he won a number of awards in white-water canoeing, a completely unnecessary sport if you ask me, which also gave him a broad back and hands like shovels. He must have roared so loud in those rapids that the only thing he's ever cast in is Wagner." My friend casually dropped the end of his cigarette into a small bucket waiting expectantly beside his chair. "It's my own pain that makes me speak so uncharitably," he admitted, although without the slightest hint of regret. "Well, you know the crucial scene: Klingsor hurls the famous spear, Parsifal catches it in midair, the strings play on . . ."

My thoughts wandered. During my last visit to Bayreuth, *Siegfried* lasted twenty minutes longer than usual. As anyone who has been there can testify, the seats in the famous Festspielhaus must have been designed to the specific personal dimensions of Richard Wagner. If the great composer were himself resurrected and stood next to me, he would have admitted that I was taller by at least an ell, or, to put it plainly, the man would have come up to my nipples. By the end of the second act my body looked like a melting ice cube which had given up all hope of ever leaving the tray. It was then that I realized that almost all male aficionados of Wagner are small of stature, which is, incidentally, why their women always appear so imposing. Then again, perhaps I'm confusing cause and effect; perhaps these men have shrunk as a result of repeated visits to Bayreuth.

"Our Parsifal," Michael H. interrupted my mental digression, "is famous for insisting that a real spear actually be thrown, whether he's singing here in Munich or at the Met. Of course there are countless ways of solving the problem with lighting or special effects, all very convincing. To resort to naturalism when it comes to spear throwing is idiotic: at best it will look ridiculous, and at worst the house will wind up with astronomical liability payments. But our Parsifal is so proud of his physical prowess, that he refuses to perform unless his opponent actually hurls the holy spear. On top of all this, it turns out that our Parsifal can't stomach our Klingsor. Probably because they've appeared opposite each other too many times; you know how stage roles frequently carry over into the private lives of the performers. 'Don't worry,' Parsifal assured me over the phone during our preliminary discussions, 'I'll catch the spear. Of course that's assuming your Klingsor is actually able to throw the damn thing, and not into the house, either.'"

"And how did Klingsor react to the challenge?"

Michael H. just sighed, so I immediately replenished his glass and lit another cigarette.

"Klingsor went completely stiff when I told him about Parsifal's demands—or I should say, even more stiff than usual. He was just finishing up some medicine-ball training with the chorus singers—incidentally, they had all agreed to meet Kundry for some aquajogging, but I'm jumping ahead of myself—and was in the middle of a deep-breathing exercise he calls 'The Five Tibetans,' when I burst in with Parsifal's demands."

I still couldn't imagine how all these confusing details were leading to my friend's white collar, but the excitement in his face persuaded me to hold my questions. But since the tale promised to be a long one, I treated my lower back to a quick program of contract and release.

He went on to tell me how a plot was hatched that evening, over aquajogging, in which Kundry begged Klingsor, still rigid with indignation, to accept Parsifal's challenge and work secretly on developing a powerful spear throw. The fight choreographer agreed to help him. For her part, Kundry was evidently still smarting from a painful affair with Parsifal at La Scala some years before. And since opera theaters around the globe were always throwing the two of them together, she was often made to suffer the added injury of Parsifal turning his back to her during their great love scene—despite any and all direction to the contrary. It seems he was also wont to walk downstage and hold his note just long enough for her to run out of breath.

"If only we had known," said Michael H., by now quite agitated. "If only the fight choreographer had mentioned something, none of this would have happened. But as it turned out, Klingsor was suddenly obsessed both with Kundry *and* with spear throwing. He went to a sporting goods store and bought a leather sports girdle. Then he went to a video shop and bought a video of the last Olympic javelin competition. Our fight choreographer supplied him with some spears out of our storage. The man knew he had only three days to practice before Parsifal arrived from the Salzburg Easter Festival to join the rehearsals."

I'd never heard of a leather sports girdle. Although since my last birthday I am the proud owner of a form-fitting, anatomically adjustable back support bandage for men. The woman who gave it to me confided that she

wore a similar model, except hers was green, with a double hook-and-eye fastener on both sides and contoured
padding. But a leather sports girdle?

"It strengthens the lower back," my friend said, a trifle
impatiently. "I have it right there in the wardrobe, along
with the two-piece lumbar support strap for preventing
painful back rotations, the adjustable inner sole for stabi-
lizing the ankle, the active elbow bandage, and much
more. Much more. I'd be happy to let you take anything
you could use, but I'm not sure we won't be needing them;
after all, the performance has only been *postponed*."

No sooner had the first full rehearsal begun than disaster struck. Amfortas, bent on playing his wound, kept
doubling over very dramatically, clutching the blood-
stained cloth covering his groin, until a mighty attack of
pain in the middle of a glissando sent his voice soaring
from C-sharp into a register matched only by a true cas-
trato. Fortunately the props crew had set out a stretcher,
since one was called for at this point in the opera, so the
paramedics were able to carry the victim quickly offstage.
Nevertheless, because these men had trouble distinguish-
ing between art and reality, they began to treat the blood-
stained groin area, which led to further complications
that my friend only hinted at.

The rest of the rehearsal was no less eventful: when
Klingsor made his entrance he was carrying not just one
spear, but five. And judging by his unsteady carriage, he
must have taken a few nips beforehand to bolster his
courage; in any case, he immediately started firing off his
weapons, eyes flashing, without waiting for the orchestra's

entrance, so that he seemed less the embodiment of a medieval hero than an antiaircraft battery from World War II. After the fourth throw, however, it became apparent that Klingsor had overestimated his physical capabilities; all of a sudden he clutched his back, dropped to his knees, and collapsed with a light groan over his last spear, in precisely the same place on stage where King Amfortas had been wounded a few minutes prior.

Nor was Parsifal spared. When the first two spears came flying his way, he plucked them from the air as if he were picking cherries from a tree. By the third throw his face was showing a mixture of strain and excitement. He began anxiously clenching and unclenching his famous fists. When Klingsor threw his fourth, it was all he could do to bat it away; not even his opponent's obvious distress seemed to give him any satisfaction.

At that moment Kundry walked on—"No, 'walked on' doesn't do it justice," my friend corrected himself: "The woman stormed on stage like some Greek goddess of revenge and demanded to play the love scene with Parsifal right then and there. Naturally this ran contrary to the rehearsal plan."

And the conductor allowed it?

"With both Amfortas and Klingsor out of commission he didn't have much choice. Besides, he was excited to see our Kundry in such an obvious state of arousal. You know the scene, right?"

"Parsifal saves himself by thinking about his mother?"— I was grateful that the exam hadn't been much harder.

"She tries to seduce him into kissing her," my friend

confirmed, "and to do so she bends her body back like a reed swaying in the wind."

"And he has to bend with her!" I generally consider metaphors with reeds swaying in the wind hackneyed and clichéd, but in this case the image was enlightening. Besides, I knew what was coming. I could feel it in my back. "Even Parsifal," I surmised, "even Parsifal, the champion canoeist was felled by his treacherous back."

Again I could see that Michael H. would have happily nodded in agreement, but his neck brace only allowed an approving blink.

"At that point I invited all the concerned parties over to my place. After all, as dramaturg I was partly responsible for what had happened. In my naïveté I imagined we would talk things over calmly and professionally and come to a reasonable solution. Just in case of an emergency, a pharmacist friend had equipped me with the orthopedic equipment you can see there in my wardrobe. Of course my hopes were in vain; the cast treated my apartment as just another venue for Wagnerian bickering. In the end I had to put my foot down."

I knew my talented friend was capable of many things, but of putting his foot down? Some men like nothing better than putting down their feet, but those tend to become directors and wear scarves around their necks. Dramaturgs, I thought, achieve their greatness by way of their sensitivity, even self-doubt. Perhaps they should all be advised to wear a neck brace as part of their professional uniform.

My friend read my thoughts. "Now you know. That's

exactly how it happened. They had jointly agreed that I was the one to blame for their collective misfortune, and I was outraged. I had to put my foot down. But in putting down my foot, I flung up my arm, and *voilà!*" Here he tapped his empty wineglass against his neck brace. "At least Klingsor was kind enough to call for an ambulance."

Out on the street a drunken sailor tossed two streamers right in front of my nose.

Twenty-first Vertebra

THE TORTOISE

I guess we started talking about turtles because of Lena's heavy back-pack. These days small children are taught the serious meaning of life less by means of strict moral preachings and more through the leaden weight of their satchels. When my daughter leaves for school in the morning, she looks like a charming primordial reptile which some lovesick paleontologist has adorned with a red cap and a green tassel. Or else like an astronaut who has to carry enough oxygen for several moon walks in an algae-colored backpack, although moon-walkers have an easier time moving around.

"The turtle's shell," said Lena, who could imitate her biology teacher so well you felt he was sitting right at the table with you, "and please note that this applies to tortoises as well as sea turtles, did not develop because the animal had to protect itself from predators—everyone knows what those are, right?—from its natural enemies who were swimming ferociously through the ocean or hunting fiercely on dry land. The shell is actually a further development of their backbone."

"Lena, please, eat your noodles," her mother said when she saw that my professional curiosity was threatening to disrupt the Master Parental Plan. "If they get cold you'll like them even less."

Our daughter took her fork and, unmoved by her mother's request, constructed a small tower of pasta. "You know, once upon a time they didn't even have a shell, but then they needed a stronger backbone for their muscles, or else they wouldn't be able to swim anymore and would all drown."

Her repeated mention of a backbone did away with any and all parental plans. "Why wouldn't they have been able to swim anymore?" I asked impatiently. "And besides, why should a turtle want to swim in the first place?"

"Because of its *muscles*, of course," she answered with amazing self-assurance. "Our teacher told us that all *higher* forms of life have muscles that are designed to work closely together with backbones and spinal cords. You of all people should be able to understand that, right?" Only an eleven-year-old can look her father in the eye so knowingly.

"Do you know why *most* men walk crooked?" I attempted to defend myself: "In some cases it's because they're so stressed by their work; and in others it's because they carried their daughter piggyback too many times." As soon as I said that I realized it was a mistake.

"And what about women?" Lena fought back. "Aren't they stressed by their work? I don't see Claudia Schiffer walking around all hunched over."

Maybe it was a big mistake to agree to let my daughter go to a daycare center founded by a gang of male feminists who were fed up with traditional gender roles. On the other hand, I did appreciate her choice of a role model— if not for the same reasons.

"You better start working more closely together with your noodles," Lena's mother interjected. "And even if you aren't a turtle, you should still eat your lettuce." Then she turned to me: "Perhaps you delve into all the biological nuances later on tonight. After she finishes her homework and practices her gymnastics."

Lena's mother, I thought on my way to my workroom above the garage, is truly touching in her efforts to insure that not one of our child's talents remains undeveloped. In a few years I'll have a daughter who can recite Horace in the original as she leaps onto a flying trapeze. Then on her way down, in the middle of a double salto, she can discourse the secrets of photosynthesis or the evolution of the Galapagos tortoise. It's not that I'm afraid of her turning into Superwoman: it's just that I'm sad I won't be able to catch her anymore when she lands. And I'm worried that, as a result, in her eyes I might become an old fart. The closest I've come to gymnastics is watching it on TV. And whenever it comes on I quickly change the channel and pretend that I can't stomach the frozen smiles and garish costumes. In reality I'm simply bothered by the contrast between my own pitiful kneebends, secretly performed beside my desk, and the dishearteningly limber teenagers on the screen.

To console myself I keep a secret file of press clippings on athletic injuries, all carefully sorted by event and disability. For days following a tennis tournament, a gymnastic competition, or a ski event I am often occupied with updating my collection. Because the sports industry is always inventing new ways to strain ligaments, tear muscles, and crush vertebrae, my archive is growing by leaps and bounds, so to speak. Unfortunately I have yet to find a soulmate who shares my secret passion. Maybe I should take out a personals ad.

"So, the thing with the turtles is this," said Lena, who suddenly materialized next to my desk. "Over time they got bigger and bigger and heavier and heavier. And they used to swim with their vertebrae. Not with their arms and legs like we do, but more like fish, you know. And because they grew so heavy and overweight, their back had to grow stronger. Then one day it got all crusted over, and suddenly the turtle had a shell. Then their backbone became a round hard plate. And now the animal can't swim anymore, just paddle, and nobody knows what's going to happen next, not even our teacher. But somebody better do something soon or else it'll be too late."

Lena was born in Vienna, and she shares the apocalyptic mentality for which the inhabitants of that city are famous. Even my careful attempts to clarify the passage of time involved in the evolutionary process were not enough to calm her down.

"They could all drown overnight because of their thick shell!" she cried. "Imagine, an entire species going kaput just like that!"

That evening I told my daughter a bedtime story that contained only elves and fairies, two cheerful species, neither one, to my knowledge, in danger of sudden extinction. But no sooner had I tucked her in, kissed her, and turned off the light than my own thoughts once again turned to turtles and their crusty shells.

"Do you think nature resorts to metaphors?" I asked my life companion, who had completed a second dissertation on the biodiversity of small butterflies and who therefore ought to have an answer. "Do you think it's possible that nature sometimes sends us coded messages?"

My life companion looked up from her book. For several years neither one of us has had much time to read, and this particular book seemed particularly thrilling. Which is probably why her counterquestion sounded so brusque: "Do you have a problem, or are you just trying to solve a crossword puzzle?"

The phrase "Do you have a problem?"—along with the word "kafkaesque"—figured high on the list of expressions we had sworn never to use. We made that oath over breakfast after our first night together. But now that my life was rapidly becoming kafkaesque, I forgot all about our vow.

"It's about the turtles," I said hesitantly. "More precisely, about their shells. After what Lena told me I can't get rid of the feeling that these reptiles are trying to send me a message. Nothing very specific, just a vague kind of hint. Something to do with where our own backs are headed . . ."

"You realize of course that turtles have a ventral plastron as well as a dorsal carapace," Delia interrupted. "In other words, they have shells on the front as well as the back," she explained. "And this is true whether you're talking about the cryptodira or the pleurodira."

I was moved by the care she showed these taxonomic distinctions and begged her to go on.

"Turtles are categorized into different suborders according to how they retract their heads. The hidden-necked turtles pull them straight back, while the side-necked ones simply turn them whenever threatened."

Now I felt an even closer relationship to the reptile. Apparently in ancient times it had developed highly advanced defense mechanisms. Never again would I gaze upon a turtle with my earlier indifference.

"And what do we know about their gender-specific behavior?"

"The physical work is taken care of by the females, of course," answered my life companion coolly. "They're the ones who shovel the sand over the freshly laid eggs, while the exhausted male hangs around and waits. Was that what you were thinking of when you were asking about metaphors?" She picked up her marker and highlighted a sentence in her book.

There are certain deep philosophical questions that can be made to sound ridiculous by an overly precise answer. I confess: during our last vacation I had refused to build a sand castle for Lena. Not only because I consider them pitifully bourgeois, but also because I was loyally following my doctor's strict orders not to heave, shove, or toss anything with a shovel. However, Lena insisted on her castle, and her mother wound up doing all the work until, overcome with shame, I finally pitched in.

Was Delia referring to this? Or was her barb meant to dig even deeper?

"It could be," I said, refusing to let myself be cowed into silence by her book. "At least it's theoretically possible that nature might develop one species in such a way as to send a message to a different species. And it's true that whenever my back starts hurting, I can't stop thinking about shells. My back muscles stiffen into cartilage and bone plates and I feel like an endangered crustacean. You realize that we experience our greatest sensitivity in moments of pain. And my empathy is such that in the course of a few minutes I experience the entire evolutionary history of the turtle—or really the tortoise, since I don't paddle so much as crawl. The upright gait is, as Lena would say, kaput. Chances are, any day now, I, too, will retract my head—only as a gesture, I mean—either by bringing it straight back or turning it in, depending on what kind of threat I'm facing."

"Your forebears had their reasons for learning to move upright on two legs; after all, every other animal in the African savannah could run at least twice as fast as they could"—my life companion didn't look up from her book, which, incidentally, dealt with witch cults in the Middle Ages—"and I'm sure you realize the difference between empathetic sensitivity and plain old run-of-the-mill self-pity."

What I should have realized by then was that this was not the evening to pit my impromptu theorizing against a well-polished anthropological position. But the idea wouldn't let go of me, so I blundered ahead, blithely ignoring all the fundamental, unwritten laws of matrimonial harmony.

"But what if *they* were wrong, and the turtles are right? I cried out, exacerbated. "After all, they've had their shells a lot longer than we've been walking upright. It's just as likely that our forebears, as you call them, made a mistake when they reared up on their hind legs and started to run. Maybe our so-called upright gait is nothing more than an anatomical anomaly. When eighty percent of all men can no longer walk straight, maybe it's time to recognize that we made an evolutionary mistake. The sooner we admit it, the better for all concerned."

My life companion marked her page and closed her book. "I'd really like to finish this chapter," she said. "Your pills are in the medicine cabinet. Why don't you look in on me again before you go to bed?"

That night I dreamed of soft fleshy parts over which a glittering shell was smoothly opening and closing.

The pet-store owners Havliczek & Bissinger heartily approved of my decision to give my daughter a small tortoise for her birthday. "They cost very little to maintain and nevertheless make very loyal pets," Bissinger remarked happily as he lifted the creature from its cage. "They can put up with a lot, and they are surprisingly mobile," Havliczek added, as he wrote out the bill. "I'm sure your daughter will be very delighted."

144

Twenty-second Vertebra

THE SEDUCER

My mountain climbing partner, Thekla, never complains about anything—except about men who whine about their aches and pains. We had been trekking all morning, and I was completely exhausted, so we plopped down at a small country inn. It turned out that the place was hosting a local folk dance festival, replete with all manner of yodels and shrieks and people leaping and twirling their skirts.

I had risked broaching an interesting topic in the history of medicine and religion, in the hope that it was far enough from any explicit complaint that Thekla might deign to respond. Her aversion to physical complaints stemmed from an almost fanatical stoicism, a kind of transcendental disregard for her own body—or anyone else's.

As soon as I mentioned the word "vertebrae" I could tell Thekla was beginning to suspect my motives. I was about to change the subject when a man wearing a top hat and tails walked up to us and gave a slight bow: "I couldn't help overhearing that you question the very existence of the spine." Without waiting for a reply he brushed his tails aside and, gently lifting his hat to Thekla, sat down beside her: "That happens to be of professional interest to me. With your permission, I'd be delighted to join you for a moment." Thekla, who is very polite but a little sensitive to smells, inched discreetly toward the open window.

"I never questioned its existence," I said, "any more than I question the existence of the Garmisch Folk Dance Club that was just jumping around here. I was merely saying that eighteenth-century medicine was right to distinguish between 'true' and 'false' vertebrae. In those days the cervical and lumbar vertebrae were considered 'true,' whereas the twelve thoracic ones were considered 'false.' Now, I'd be the first to question whether lumbar vertebrae really deserve to be called true, but at least they're true to their name, *vertebra*, which is to say they turn—as you perhaps know, the Latin *vertere* means 'to turn.' The only really false ones are the sacrum and the coccyx."

Thekla put her hand over her ears: "Could we please change the subject?"

The stranger was about to say something when the waitress arrived with our coffee. She, too, seemed to have noticed a strong odor and, in fact, ended up holding her little nose as she left. On stage another folk group was taking up its position.

"Perhaps," said the stranger, "you would prefer to discuss the dancing? About the pagan origins of what we have just witnessed, the vestiges of ancient fertility rites." At this point he was focused intently on Thekla's discreet décolletage and let his eyes crawl slowly up her neck until they met her own. I noticed Thekla turning slightly red, and I looked away.

Despite her obvious embarrassment, she counterattacked at once. Staring at his top hat, she said, "I didn't realize they were planning a carnival sideshow as well. Do you do magic tricks, or are you just the barker?"

But the stranger didn't respond. Still staring at Thekla's eyes, he seemed lost in thought. "Ah, the Bacchic rites, those were fun times," he said to himself, "but alas, *sic transit gloria mundi.*"

Now he was really getting on my nerves. The idea of spending the next hour in the company of a sleazy amateur magician trying to impress every woman he meets with a few Latin clichés was unbearable. In any event, with Thekla he was barking up the wrong tree: she couldn't stand "smooth-talking overeducated showoffs" any more than she could men who constantly complained about their backs.

So I was a little surprised she didn't get up and demand we leave immediately—particularly because by then even I was beginning to be bothered by the man's peculiar cologne, which seemed to have more than a hint of sulphur. But maybe Thekla was simply taking pity on my feet; after all, she was the one who insisted we climb all the way back down instead of taking the funicular—and despite all my doctor's warnings, I had agreed.

I turned away to watch a new group from the eastern Tirol which had just begun performing. The men were all dressed in lederhosen, which are so stiff you have to climb into them. Still, this particular stiffness seemed to have no effect on their dancing; they were twisting and vaulting and flinging their legs around as they swung their feathered hats with great bravado, all the while emitting a series of rutlike grunts.

Naturally that display of brute flexibility bothered me as much as the performance taking place right at my table. Not only had Thekla not done anything to get rid of the man; she was actually listening to what he was saying about snake dancing and some other pagan rites. And when the Tirolean mountain goats had finished their jumping, both Thekla and the stranger stood up and applauded!

I myself ostentatiously remained in my seat. "This kind of Saint Vitus' dance stinks if you ask me," I said, hardly masking my allusion.

"Ah!" said the stranger, turning to me as he sat back down, "that was one of my better efforts! Don't think it was easy to get *that* started at church fairs and the like. You're absolutely right, though; those people sure knew how to jump. They could really writhe about, twisting their backs into all kinds of erotic positions." Then he turned back to Thekla and said flirtatiously, "Actually the real source of *desire* is not so much the twisted back itself but the pain with which it is associated. As a good friend of mine once put it, 'We are only healed only when we learn to savor our suffering,' although I have to admit it sounds better in French."

Aaargh! Thekla knew her Proust as well as I. "A good friend of mine" indeed! Thekla could have easily unmasked our table guest for the charlatan he was, but her pale blue eyes radiated only interest and understanding and a strange sense of relief. What next? Nietzsche? No, now they had moved to Dostoyevsky and were discussing whether human consciousness was rooted in spiritual or physical suffering. Thekla said something about a "jabbing pain" she occasionally felt in her upper neck as well as a "periodic stiffness" that often attacked her shoulder. Never had she mentioned anything of the kind to me. But by that point I didn't care. I was just waiting for the stranger to claim that he had chatted with Dostoyevsky once—in Russian, of course—about the brothers Karamazov. If he did that I would stand up—perfectly cool and calm—and walk out. A big blast of oompah music announced a new performance.

Thekla seemed totally enthralled; she had placed her ear right next to the man's mouth, while he had very gently laid three slender fingers on her left hand. As soon as the music quieted down a little I heard him saying, "You would be amazed, my dear, at what pleasure and joy there can be in letting go"—and she was even smiling at the man!—"but I wanted to tell you about Dostoyevsky. Or really about his beard, it was whirled in a very bizarre way, and as he once told me, though it sounded better in Russian . . ."

I paid the bill at the counter and phoned for a taxi. I didn't see Thekla again until a month later. It was a dreary day—winter had arrived with a vengeance. In a crooked little sidestreet off the Maximilianstrasse there is a certain orthopedic undergarment shop, known to connoisseurs for its wide range of exquisite warmers made of natural fibers and specially fitted for every part of the body. The atmosphere is so discreet that even customers who have known each other for years courteously look the other way if they happen to meet at the cash register.

"One fleece-lined camisole and one eiderdown cervical pillow," the cashier remarked, then named a figure and handed the lady ahead of me a package, daintily wrapped and tied.

"Do you take credit cards?" asked the client.

"Thekla!" I cried out when I heard her voice.

A reproachful cough from the cashier reminded me I had just broken the rules.

Standing in the slush outside, I asked Thekla the question that had been bothering me for weeks: "What in the world did you find so fascinating about that clown in the top hat and tails? Was it his cologne or his formidable coccyx?"

Thekla looked at the package she was clutching in her arm. "You have no right to speak of him that way," she answered gently. "Besides, he gave me something that is bound to bring you and me closer and closer. He gave me courage and conviction, and above all, he gave me faith. He convinced me to believe in my own pain. To take it seriously, to accept it as a challenge. To ask not 'What is my back doing to me?' but 'What am I doing to my back?' Now you and I will be able to sit by the fireplace and share. We can reminisce about back clinics and automatic stair climbers. About true and false vertebrae. About our spinal sins and their absolution . . ."

I realized then and there that another sufferer had been unleashed upon the world.

A light snow was falling. Without saying a word, I embraced my new comrade in pain, tenderly, gingerly. High overhead, the street lamp flickered on—a quiet signal of redeeming hope.

Twenty-third Vertebra

BACK IN THE SADDLE AGAIN

My American translator and I knew each other only by transatlantic phone and fax, and when I found out that I had to travel to New York on business, I immediately let him know, so that we could arrange a meeting. "Listen," he suggested, "why don't you come on down for a visit?"

For a few seconds I pondered the possible meaning of "come on down"—a newcomer to my English vocabulary—but when he mentioned his wife's name, it sounded reassuringly European, and I felt safe enough to accept his invitation.

Only when I started talking to my travel agent did I appreciate the weakness of my grasp of North American geography. I knew my translator lived somewhere outside Houston, but I had no idea how far apart New York and Texas really were. However, my curiosity quickly overcame my hesitation, and I had the agent book a flight. As usual, I decided to pay a little more for a seat in business class: experience has taught me that the additional cost is nothing compared to the price my back would pay for a seat in economy.

On the way down I sat next to a chiropractor who was returning from Russia; he was apparently part of a whole group who had gone there to spread the good word concerning chiropractic. Dr. B. explained to me the history of this therapy in the United States, which seemed to consist mostly of an ongoing struggle with the American Medical Association, which had, as he put it "conspired to put us out of business."

He went on to describe the concept as he had learned it at the Logan College of Chiropractic in St. Louis. In actuality it differed very little from other methods of physical therapy, except in the importance it ascribed to "spinal adjustments"—specially applied pushes and pulls designed to bring the spinal column into proper alignment, and thereby rid the body of damaging tension, as well as its worst symptom, pain. Certain schools of chiropractic, it turned out, "especially one up in Minnesota," go so far as to apply this treatment to such seemingly unrelated problems as chronic sinusitis. (Here I made a mental note to ask my translator about the exact geographic location of Minnesota.)

"Just like anything else," Dr. B. explained, "some people go a little too far. But I'll tell you, I adjust my kids' backs twice a week and they have fewer colds than anybody in the whole school."

I was about to launch into my own experience with spinal adjustments—which was certainly no worse than with other physical therapies—when the flight attendant gently prepared the business passengers for landing by offering another drink.

My translator met me at the gate. As a rule, translators are not a feast for the eye. Years of underpaid and mostly unrecognized labor for undeserving authors and mindless publishing houses tend to take their toll. The poor souls are typically hunched over, prone to quibble over archaic usages, and often reduced to sighing at their cruel fate.

Thus I was pleasantly surprised to meet a totally different specimen. My translator was tall and blond, his hairline ran high, and his demeanor was decidedly sunny. During my whole stay, he made not a single pedantic reference. As we drove to his home, he informed me that he had concocted a program to give me a taste of the "Lone Star State"; since I was only able to spare a day and a half he said it would be what he called a whirlwind tour. But first he graciously allowed me to take a much needed nap.

Before dinner we sat down to work over a very cold beer.

"You know," he explained, "the greatest difficulty I'm having is with the constant play on words. Take *Kreuz*, for example: in German it can mean both a cross and the small of the back, and you have this ongoing leitmotiv of bearing the cross. Or else *Wirbel*: I can say 'backbone' or 'spine,' but nothing that conveys the idea of 'whirlwind,' which is of course the same word in German. And only someone well versed in Latin will see the connection between 'vertebra,' 'vortex,' and 'vertigo,' and that would be pretty heavy-handed anyway."

All I could do was agree, and be glad that I wasn't a translator.

"And the worst thing," he added, "is that until now I've always been an advocate of the empathic imagination as the key to translating literature. But this is the last time I'm doing a book like this. When I finished the chapter on Tarzan I started having to spend thirty minutes a day stretching before I sat down at my desk, and by the time I reached 'Ski Jumping' I was already seeing a chiropractor."

"Was he from the Logan College of Chiropractic?" I asked and referred him to Dr. B.

After we had finished making the proper adjustments to the translation we went out to dinner at a place that claimed to serve "the best Bar-B-Que in Texas," which, my friend assured me, made it also the best in the world. I followed his example and asked for extra jalapeños. That proved a big mistake.

After I had tried to drown the explosion in my throat with more icy beer we drove outside town and headed west, passing landmark after landmark of Texas history, a field of study I had evidently grossly underestimated. Before long we seemed to be the only ones on the road not driving a pickup truck, a vehicle that would have obviously made my uncle very happy, as my translator pointed out. Although he had said we wouldn't be driving very far, it was two hours of freeway later that we pulled up in front of a dilapidated structure known as a "honky-tonk"—this particular one called itself the Watering Hole.

"A lot of Texans," my friend explained as we went in, "don't tend to believe in psychosomatic symptoms. It's one thing if you get hurt in a fight or get thrown off a horse like my mother did once, but the idea that your back, or anything else, could be sore because of something you're repressing—they'd just call that a lot of psychological bullshit. And even if you run into somebody who's so bent over you know he's in pain—well, I really wouldn't try talking to him about denial."

"Inside" was really still outside: the honky-tonk consisted of a number of tables and benches underneath a kind of roof without walls. A man sitting by a big box came up to us and said something I couldn't quite make out: two minutes later he brought us each a bottle of some local beer—once again exceedingly chilled.

"You boys are in for a treat tonight," he said—by now I was beginning to understand. "Cause tonight we got Ed Bob Cohen and his Horned Toad Band."

My friend answered my puzzled look with a detailed zoological description of the lizard known as the "horned toad." "Except that here we pronounce it 'horny' toad, so that the name of the band is really an untranslatable pun."

Just then there was some commotion by the big box of frozen beer, and in walked four exceedingly scraggly musicians with long hair and beards, and another dressed in a light-colored western-styled suit with bolo tie. All were wearing what I assumed to be Stetson hats.

The entire Watering Hole—about a hundred cowboys and cowgirls—stood up and started cheering and waving their hats. Within a few minutes Ed Bob Cohen and his Horned Toad Band had the entire honky-tonk on their feet. A man neither one of us had ever laid eyes on bought our whole table another round.

Several dances later, a whole chorus of honky-tonkers started shouting "Cotton-eyed Joe! Cotton-eyed Joe!" and everyone began shoving the tables off to one side.

It all happened so quickly, and the din was so enormous that my translator didn't even try to explain what was going on. Before I knew it two women wearing western boots and shirts and jeans had grabbed me by either arm and pulled me into a line of people who were beginning to stomp to what was evidently a very popular tune. Ed Bob broke out his fiddle and suddenly the whole line skipped forward three or four times and everybody kicked up their legs as high as possible and shouted "Bull-shit!" then walked back three steps, shouted "Bull-shit!" one more time, and started the whole thing all over again.

"You drunk or something?" one of the women asked me. As soon as I opened my mouth she realized she was dealing with a foreigner, "a real foreigner," as she put it, not just somebody from out of state. "Well, we'll just have to show you how to dance the Cotton-eyed Joe. When I slap you on the ass, you kick up your legs like everybody else." We skipped forward again, the whole line swung up its leg, and she slapped me exactly as promised. I felt the pain flaring up, but then I too kicked my leg high in the air and shouted "Bull-shit!" as loudly as I could. To my amazement the pain subsided, I felt younger by years, and continued to dance the Cotton-eyed Joe for another half hour.

Three days later, back home in Munich, I unwrapped the package my translator had given me as a memento of my time in Texas. There was a bottle of hot sauce and a compact disc. My friend had written a dedication on the hot sauce: "Good for what ails you—try it on your back sometime." The CD cover sported a picture of a horned toad wearing a bolo tie and a Stetson.

At the slightest sign of stiffening I now put on Ed Bob full volume, kick my legs up as high as they'll go, and shout "Bull-*shit!*" at the top my lungs. The hot sauce remains unopened.

Twenty-fourth Vertebra

GOODBYE

"So, subjectively speaking, do you feel better now?" asked my psychotherapist when I told her I had finished my book. A few months before I would have answered her snidely that my feelings were always "subjective"—but writing the book had kept Pain away for so long that I was in a pretty good mood. So good, in fact, that this was our last scheduled session.

"I'll have to wait and see," I said. "At the moment I'm not complaining. But the true test won't come until the book appears on the market. You can't imagine the spasms a pan from a major paper can cause."

"*Book* and *back*," she said, "that's interesting. They even sound alike, and both have a spine. Have you frequently connected the two in your dreams?"

Recently my psychotherapist and I have been sitting opposite each other in what she calls "a slightly modified position," so that we both can maintain an alert and unobstructed free flow of associations. Supposedly Freud himself suggested this arrangement—I'm not familiar with the appropriate passage. However, I did once have to lie down on his famous couch for a documentary film on the fiftieth anniversary of his death, and I can say from experience that Freud was either a genuine sadist or else prolapsed discs were less common in his day than hysteria. This poorly upholstered, sagging piece of furniture with its pseudo-oriental pattern is absolute murder on the sensitive spine. But perhaps it was really designed to force the patient into a posture of submission, a physical emblem of symbolic ego restraint—if so, there's nothing better suited than a sagging couch with broken springs.

"Or maybe a bed of nails," I quietly intoned. In one chapter for this book (which I eventually cut), I started to analyze the relationship between back pain and various world religions. My friend Nasrin gave me some wonderful tidbits, such as the Arabic greeting "*Tasim*," which means "I bow down to you." It turns out that the world of the crescent moon is none too easy on the crooked back. Not that other religious communities are any better, which is why the chapter had to go: too much material can pose as great an obstacle to the writer as too little.

"Did you just say 'bed of nails'? Were you thinking of your critics?" asked the therapist gently but resolutely.

"Not at all," I answered hastily. "I don't think the critics are going to respond to this book one way or the other, which is all right with me. After all, I'm not trying to write the novel of the century. I'm sure there'll be those who point out that Dante's portrayal of backs in pain was a lot more grotesque, and others who fault me for not being postmodern enough. And invariably someone will ob-ject that he or she had a totally different experience in Taipei. Besides, I won't believe it's out until I see it on the shelves; after all, a number of journals didn't consider the subject 'current enough' when I offered them serial rights, and some editors never even acknowledged receipt of my manuscript."

My therapist suddenly looked worried. Staring out the window, she asked, "Have you ever considered that you might have some kind of messianic complex? Or that you might think of yourself as a male Cassandra, an unrecognized but persecuted seer? That would be per-fectly understandable, given what you've been through in the past few years."

I had never heard my therapist talk this way. Until now all she had done was guide me to understand what *I* might have inflicted on my back, not the other way around. I looked at the therapist framed by the win-dow, against the dreary background of the vacant lot outside.

"Maybe I have become a little oversensitive," I admit-ted. "After all, the pain's practically gone, but I keep hav-ing these annoying associations. Just yesterday, when my father spoke to me about the curved shape of the uni-verse, all I could think about was my new cummerbund. Even now, looking out the window, I didn't think to my-self 'landscape' or 'vacant lot.' I thought '*back-*ground'— 'what a painfully dreary background.'"

The therapist crossed her legs. "Are you trying to say that your entire perception has shifted? That you believe your problems with your spine are now in your head? Could it be that you're substituting a feeling of professional frustration for the physical pain you no longer feel? Think about your irrational hatred of critics, for example. Have you gotten so used to the condition of being hurt that you actually *need* pain to maintain a complete sense of identity?"

I kept staring out the window. In mind games like this the patient never has a chance.

"Can't I have my cake and hate it too?" I asked anyway. "Can't I get rid of my back pain without losing my loathing for dumb critics?"

My therapist cleared her throat. I thought I detected a hint of reproach.

"You have to understand," she said quickly, "you've been in terrible pain for years. Sometimes you used to hobble in here like you were on your last legs. Your whole life seemed as bent out of shape as your back. Yesterday, when I was looking over your files, it dawned on me how in everything you talked about, whether it was your work or ski jumping or sex or your old car—you invariably detected an enemy. But an enemy for which you were always a match—never once did you admit defeat. I don't know the latest medical report on your spine, but from my point of view, as far as your spirit is concerned, you are a genuine hero."

No one, and I mean no one, had spoken so encouragingly to me in ages. I was used to being reproached about my lifestyle, warned to take things easier, to move more efficiently, to behave with greater moral rectitude. But not once had anyone included an encouraging word of praise. I alone had had to bear this burden of my original sin. There was no Eve to share the weight, no Satan. And now, suddenly: redemption.

But as soon as I received the redeeming words of recognition, I felt myself strangely alone. In fact, I felt a new defense bubbling up defiantly inside me. I began to suspect my therapist of doing something I would never have thought her capable of, namely a so-called paradoxical intervention. Let me give an example of this therapeutic strategy: a doctor has a patient who thinks he's Napoleon. The clever therapist doesn't contradict the man; instead, he expresses his most heartfelt condolences for the defeat at Waterloo and talks sympathetically about the high incidence of stomach pain among great world leaders. If all goes well, the patient comes to consider his doctor schizophrenic and himself a specialist in that disorder, at which point he is effectively cured.

Was my therapist glorifying me in order to make clear to me the absurdity of my complaints? Or was she worried I was drifting into a full-blown persecution mania featuring a cast of well-known critics and had decided I was better off focused on my back? Or maybe she had mixed feelings about losing me as a patient?

The dreary sky held out no answer. The silence spread, and I ruminated on my original sin.

"I've never talked about Eve, because back pain is such a male problem," I said finally. "Because I'm convinced that only those women who consciously or unconsciously carry—"

"That's the first time you've ever mentioned any Eve," my therapist interjected. "And when you say 'carry,' maybe you're seeing yourself as a kind of Christopher? Bearing the Messiah on your back, across the hostile torrents of criticism?"

"I've never talked about Eve," I repeated, "because I'm convinced that only those women who consciously or unconsciously carry themselves like men suffer from these symptoms, which weren't designed for them. A man has to protect his private parts—that's why hunching forward evolved into a natural male instinct. Naturally women, too, have to protect their reproductive parts, but the closed legs of the female are better designed for that purpose than the male hunch. Men without this instinct are absolutely helpless against a well-aimed kick in the groin. Like so many human problems, back pain simply serves as a reminder that we are an advanced life form."

The therapist opened the window, always a reliable sign that the session was nearly at an end. "Are you still afraid of those women you described as 'strong' and with whom you seem unable to cope except in your writing?"

A cold draft on my back silenced me for a moment. I thought about Antje and Daphne, about Keto and Ursel, Barbara and Sara. The fragrant drizzle outside filled me with a feeling of yearning and imminent farewell.

"You know," I said, standing up, "this really has helped my *iliolumbalis*. And you're absolutely right to tell me not to take the critics so seriously."

We both stood by the door a moment, poised in reflection.

"But what I'm most grateful for," I continued, "is that I've finally come to recognize my true calling."

"And what is that?"

"Complaining."

My therapist smiled. "Well, then, maybe the therapy really did do you some good." We shook hands and said goodbye.